Cancer

Recent Titles in
Q&A Health Guides

Bipolar Disorder: Your Questions Answered
Victor B. Stolberg

Schizophrenia: Your Questions Answered
Romeo Vitelli

Gender Identity and Expression: Your Questions Answered
M. Killian Kinney

Cancer

Your Questions Answered

Lara Thompson

BLOOMSBURY ACADEMIC
NEW YORK • LONDON • OXFORD • NEW DELHI • SYDNEY

BLOOMSBURY ACADEMIC
Bloomsbury Publishing Inc, 1359 Broadway, New York, NY 10018, USA
Bloomsbury Publishing Plc, 50 Bedford Square, London, WC1B 3DP, UK
Bloomsbury Publishing Ireland, 29 Earlsfort Terrace, Dublin 2, D02 AY28, Ireland

BLOOMSBURY, BLOOMSBURY ACADEMIC and the Diana logo are trademarks of Bloomsbury Publishing Plc

First published in the United States of America 2026

A catalog record for this book is available from the Library of Congress.

ISBN: HB: 979-8-7651-2098-9
ePDF: 979-8-7651-2100-9
eBook: 979-8-7651-2099-6

Series: Q&A Health Guides

Typeset by Integra Software Services Pvt. Ltd.
Printed and bound in the United States of America

For product safety related questions contact productsafety@bloomsbury.com.

To find out more about our authors and books visit www.bloomsbury.com and sign up for our newsletters.

This book is dedicated to my dad, John Wendt, whose cancer experience taught me not only about the disease and its physical impact, but also about grit and grace.

Contents

Series Foreword

All of us have questions about our health. Is this normal? Should I be doing something differently? Whom should I talk to about my concerns? And our modern world is full of answers. Thanks to the internet, there's a wealth of information at our fingertips, from forums where people can share their personal experiences to Wikipedia articles to the full text of medical studies. But finding the right information can be an intimidating and difficult task—some sources are written at too high a level, others have been oversimplified, while still others are heavily biased or simply inaccurate.

Q&A Health Guides address the needs of readers who want accurate, concise answers to their health questions, authored by reputable and objective experts, and written in clear and easy-to-understand language. This series focuses on the topics that matter most to young adult readers, including various aspects of physical and emotional well-being as well as other components of a healthy lifestyle. These guides will also serve as a valuable tool for parents, school counselors, and others who may need to answer teens' health questions.

All books in the series follow the same format to make finding information quick and easy. Each volume begins with an essay on health literacy and why it is so important when it comes to gathering and evaluating health information. Next, the top five myths and misconceptions that surround the topic are dispelled. The heart of each guide is a collection of questions and answers, organized thematically. A selection of five case studies provides real-world examples to illuminate key concepts. Rounding out each volume are a directory of resources, glossary, and index. It is our hope that the books in this series will not only provide valuable information but will also help guide readers toward a lifetime of healthy decision-making.

Acknowledgments

Thank you to my husband, Nathan, who sweetly believes that now that I have published a book, I'm practically JK Rowling and should be dashing off a bestseller every year from now on. It's hard to roll my eyes at someone who believes in me that much, but I manage.

Thank you to my dad and sister who looked at everything I wrote to make sure it was remotely readable. "This paragraph made me sleepy" is the best editing note I have ever gotten. And thank you to my kids and their families, who brought me cool tech and grandkids depending on what I needed that day.

Thank you to Dr. Friedman and all of my dad's incredibly professional and personable medical providers for being the kinds of people who make their patients feel heard and whole.

Thank you to my editor, Maxine Taylor, for her optimism in thinking of me for this project, and reassuring me that my lack of medical background would not be an obstacle. I've never been published in book form before and she knew this. She appealed to my vanity and pressed her advantage.

And finally, thank you to you, the reader, for your time and interest.

Introduction

Cancer is a complex topic, and one that affects nearly everyone, either directly or indirectly. One in five people worldwide will develop cancer in their lifetime, and its effects ripple outward, touching families, communities, and health care systems. Because of its impact, cancer can still feel overwhelming to talk about. The questions are hard, and the answers are often too technical or too simplified to be helpful.

I hope this book can do even a little bit to change that.

Whether you are a student, someone considering a medical career, or just seeking clarity after cancer has touched your life, these questions and answers are here to inform and empower. From the basics of cancer biology, causes and prevention, from diagnosis to treatment, and ongoing research, I hope you find approachable science-based explanations.

This is also an invitation to take a more active role in your health, by staying informed and making better decisions. Because the best way to stop cancer is to prevent anyone from getting it in the first place.

And keep in mind that while this book provides helpful and up-to-date information, it is meant for educational purposes only. It is not a substitute for professional medical advice. Always consult a qualified health care provider about any questions you have concerning your health.

Guide to Health Literacy

On her thirteenth birthday, Samantha was diagnosed with type 2 diabetes. She consulted her mom and her aunt, both of whom also have type 2 diabetes, and decided to go with their strategy of managing diabetes by taking insulin. As a result of participating in an after-school program at her middle school that focused on health literacy, she learned that she can help manage the level of glucose in her bloodstream by counting her carbohydrate intake, following a diabetic diet, and exercising regularly. But, what exactly should she do? How does she keep track of her carbohydrate intake? What is a diabetic diet? How long should she exercise and what type of exercise should she do? Samantha is a visual learner, so she turned to her favorite source of media, YouTube, to answer these questions. She found videos from individuals around the world sharing their experiences and tips, doctors (or at least people who have "Dr." in their YouTube channel names), government agencies such as the National Institutes of Health, and even video clips from cat lovers who have cats with diabetes. With guidance from the librarian and the health and science teachers at her school, she assessed the credibility of the information in these videos and even compared their suggestions to some of the print resources that she was able to find at her school library. Now, she knows exactly how to count her carbohydrate level, how to prepare and follow a diabetic diet, and how much (and what) exercise is needed daily. She intends to share her findings with her mom and her aunt, and now she wants to create a chart that summarizes what she has learned that she can share with her doctor.

Samantha's experience is not unique. She represents a shift in our society; an individual no longer views himself or herself as a passive recipient of medical care but as an active mediator of his or her own health. However, in this era when any individual can post his or her opinions and experiences with a particular health condition online with just a few clicks or publish a memoir, it is vital that people know how to assess the credibility of health information. Gone are the days when "publishing" health information required intense vetting. The health information landscape is highly saturated, and people have innumerable sources where they can find information about practically any health topic. The sources (whether print, online, or a person) that an individual consults for health information are crucial because the accuracy and trustworthiness of the information can potentially affect his or her overall health. The ability to find, select, assess, and use health information constitutes a type of literacy—health literacy—that everyone must possess.

The Definition and Phases of Health Literacy

One of the most popular definitions for health literacy comes from Ratzan and Parker (2000), who describe health literacy as "the degree to which individuals have the capacity to obtain, process, and understand basic health information and services needed to make appropriate health decisions." Recent research has extrapolated health literacy into health literacy bits, further shedding light on the multiple phases and literacy practices that are embedded within the multifaceted concept of health literacy. Although this research has focused primarily on online health information seeking, these health literacy bits are needed to successfully navigate both print and online sources. There are six phases of health information seeking: (1) Information Need Identification and Question Formulation, (2) Information Search, (3) Information Comprehension, (4) Information Assessment, (5) Information Management, and (6) Information Use.

The first phase is the *information need identification and question formulation phase.* In this phase, one needs to be able to develop and refine a range of questions to frame one's search and understand relevant health terms. In the second phase, *information search,* one has to possess appropriate searching skills, such as using proper keywords and correct spelling in search terms, especially when using search engines and databases. It is also crucial to understand how search engines work (i.e., how search results are derived, what the order of the search results means, how to use the snippets that are provided in the search results list to select websites, and how to determine which listings are ads on a search engine results page). One also has to limit reliance on surface characteristics, such as the design of a website or a book (a website or book that appears to have a lot of information or looks aesthetically pleasant does not necessarily mean it has good information) and language used (a website or book that utilizes jargon, the keywords that one used to conduct the search, or the word "information" does not necessarily indicate it will have good information). The next phase is *information comprehension*, whereby one needs to have the ability to read, comprehend, and recall the information (including textual, numerical, and visual content) one has located from the books and/or online resources.

To assess the credibility of health information (*information assessment* phase), one needs to be able to evaluate information for accuracy, evaluate how current the information is (e.g., when a website was last updated or when a book was published), and evaluate the creators of the source—for example, examine site sponsors or type of sites (.com, .gov, .edu, or .org) or the author of a book (practicing doctor, a celebrity doctor, a patient of a specific disease, etc.) to determine the believability of the person/organization providing the information. Such credibility perceptions tend to become generalized, so they must be frequently reexamined (e.g., the belief that a specific news agency always has credible health information needs continuous vetting). One also needs to evaluate the credibility of the medium (e.g., television, internet, radio, social media, and book) and evaluate—not just accept without questioning—others' claims regarding the validity of a site, book, or other specific source of information. At this stage, one has to "make sense of information gathered from diverse sources by identifying misconceptions, main and supporting ideas, conflicting information, point of view, and biases" (American Association of School Librarians [AASL], 2009, p. 13) and conclude which sources/information are valid and accurate by using conscious strategies rather than simply using intuitive judgments or "rules of thumb." This phase is the most challenging segment of health information seeking and serves as a determinant of success (or lack thereof) in the information-seeking process. The following section on Sources of Health Information further explains this phase.

The fifth phase is *information management*, whereby one has to organize information that has been gathered in some manner to ensure easy retrieval and use in the future. The last phase is *information use*, in which one will synthesize information found across various resources, draw conclusions, and locate the answer to his or her original question and/or the content that fulfills the information need. This phase also often involves implementation, such as using the information to solve a health problem; make health-related decisions; identify and engage in behaviors that will help a person to avoid health risks; share the health information found with family members and friends who may benefit from it; and advocate more broadly for personal, family, or community health.

The Importance of Health Literacy

The conception of health has moved from a passive view (someone is either well or ill) to one that is more active and process-based (someone is working toward preventing or managing disease). Hence, the dominant focus has shifted from doctors and treatments to patients and prevention, resulting in the need to strengthen our ability and confidence (as patients and consumers of health care) to look for, assess, understand, manage, share, adapt, and use health-related information. An individual's health literacy level has been found to predict his or her health status better than age, race, educational attainment, employment status, and income level (National Network of Libraries of Medicine, 2013). Greater health literacy also enables individuals to better communicate with health care providers such as doctors, nutritionists, and therapists, as they can pose more relevant, informed, and useful questions to health care providers. Another added advantage of greater health literacy is better information-seeking skills, not only for health but also in other domains, such as completing assignments for school.

Sources of Health Information: The Good, the Bad, and the In-Between

For generations, doctors, nurses, nutritionists, health coaches, and other health professionals have been the trusted sources of health information. Additionally, researchers have found that young adults, when they have health-related questions, typically turn to a family member who has had firsthand experience with a health condition because of their family member's close proximity and because of their past experience with, and trust in, this individual. Expertise should be a core consideration when consulting a person, website, or book for health information. The credentials and background of the person or author and conflicting interests of the author (and his or her organization) must be checked and validated to ensure the likely credibility of the health information they are conveying. While books often have implied credibility because of the peer-review process involved, self-publishing has challenged this credibility, so qualifications of book authors should also be verified. When it comes to health information, currency of the source must also be examined. When examining health information/studies presented, pay attention to the exhaustiveness of research methods utilized to offer recommendations or conclusions. Small and nondiverse sample size is often—but not always—an indication of reduced credibility. Studies that confuse correlation with causation are another potential issue to watch for. Information seekers must also pay attention to the sponsors of the research studies. For example, if a study is sponsored by manufacturers of drug Y and the study recommends that drug Y is the best treatment to manage or cure a disease, this may indicate a lack of objectivity on the part of the researchers.

The internet is rapidly becoming one of the main sources of health information. Online forums, news agencies, personal blogs, social media sites, pharmacy sites, and celebrity "doctors" are all offering medical and health information targeted to various types of people in regard to all types of diseases and symptoms. There are professional journalists, citizen journalists, hoaxers, and people paid to write fake health news on various sites that may appear to have a legitimate domain name and may even have authors who claim to have professional credentials, such as an MD. All these sites *may* offer useful information or information that appears to be useful and relevant; however, much of the information may be debatable and may fall into gray areas that require readers to discern credibility, reliability, and biases.

While broad recognition and acceptance of certain media, institutions, and people often serve as the most popular determining factors to assess credibility of health information among young people, keep in mind that there are legitimate internet sites, databases, and books that publish health information and serve as sources of health information for doctors, other health sites, and members of the public. For example, MedlinePlus (https://medlineplus.gov) has trusted sources on over 975 diseases and conditions and presents the information in easy-to-understand language.

The chart here presents factors to consider when assessing credibility of health information. However, keep in mind that these factors function only as a guide and require continuous updating to keep abreast with the changes in the landscape of health information, information sources, and technologies.

The chart can serve as a guide; however, approaching a librarian about how one can go about assessing the credibility of both print and online health information is far more effective than using generic checklist-type tools. While librarians are not health experts, they can apply and teach patrons strategies to determine the credibility of health information.

With the prevalence of fake sites and fake resources that appear to be legitimate, it is important to use the following health information assessment tips to verify health information that one has obtained (St. Jean et al., 2015, p. 151):

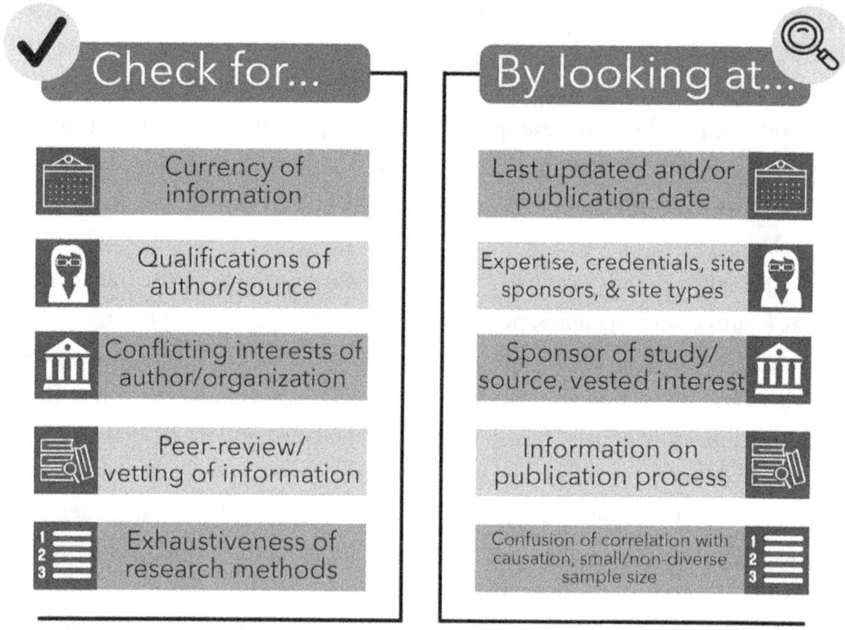

All images from flaticon.com

- **Don't assume you are right**: Even when you feel very sure about an answer, keep in mind that the answer may not be correct, and it is important to conduct (further) searches to validate the information.
- **Don't assume you are wrong**: You may actually have correct information, even if the information you encounter does not match—that is, you may be right and the resources that you have found may contain false information.
- **Take an open approach**: Maintain a critical stance by not including your preexisting beliefs as keywords (or letting them influence your choice of keywords) in a search, as this may influence what it is possible to find out.
- **Verify, verify, and verify**: Information found, especially on the internet, needs to be validated, no matter how the information appears on the site (i.e., regardless of the appearance of the site or the quantity of information that is included).

Health literacy comes with experience navigating health information. Professional sources of health information, such as doctors, health care providers, and health databases, are still the best, but one also has the power to search for health information and then verify it by consulting with these trusted sources and by using the health information assessment tips and guide shared previously.

Mega Subramaniam, PhD
Associate Professor, College of Information Studies,
University of Maryland

References and Further Reading

American Association of School Librarians (AASL). (2009). *Standards for the 21st-century learner in action.* Chicago, IL: American Association of School Librarians.

Hilligoss, B., & Rieh, S.-Y. (2008). Developing a unifying framework of credibility assessment: Construct, heuristics, and interaction in context. *Information Processing & Management, 44*(4), 1467–84.

Kuhlthau, C. C. (1988). Developing a model of the library search process: Cognitive and affective aspects. *Reference Quarterly, 28*(2), 232–42.

National Network of Libraries of Medicine (NNLM). (2013). *Health literacy.* Bethesda, MD: National Network of Libraries of Medicine. Retrieved from nnlm.gov/outreach/consumer/hlthlit.html.

Ratzan, S. C., & Parker, R. M. (2000). Introduction. In C. R. Selden, M. Zorn, S. C. Ratzan, & R. M. Parker (Eds.), *National Library of Medicine current bibliographies in medicine: Health literacy.* NLM Pub. No. CBM 2000–1. Bethesda, MD: National Institutes of Health, U.S. Department of Health and Human Services.

St. Jean, B., Subramaniam, M., Taylor, N. G., Follman, R., Kodama, C., & Casciotti, D. (2015). The influence of positive hypothesis testing on youths' online health-related information seeking. *New Library World, 116*(3/4), 136–54.

St. Jean, B., Greene Taylor, N., Kodama, C., & Subramaniam, M. (2017). Assessing the health information source perceptions of tweens using card-sorting exercises. *Journal of Information Science, 44*(2), 148–64. https://doi.org/10.1177/0165551516687728.

Subramaniam, M., St. Jean, B., Taylor, N. G., Kodama, C., Follman, R., & Casciotti, D. (2015). Bit by bit: Using design-based research to improve the health literacy of adolescents. *JMIR Research Protocols, 4*(2), paper e62. Retrieved from http://www.ncbi.nlm.nih.gov/pmc/articles/PMC4464334/.

Valenza, J. (2016). Truth, truthiness, and triangulation: A news literacy toolkit for a "post-truth" world [Web log]. November 26. Retrieved from http://blogs.slj.com/neverendingsearch/2016/11/26/truth-truthiness-triangulation-and-the-librarian-way-a-news-literacy-toolkit-for-a-post-truth-world/.

Common Misconceptions about Cancer

1. Cancer is a single disease that can appear anywhere in the body

Cancer is a comprehensive or catchall term. There are more than 200 different types and sub-types of cancers, and they are all genetically distinct from one another. When a cancer metastasizes, or spreads to another part of the body, the new tumor will be identical to the original cancer's cells. So, if a cancerous tumor in the colon spreads to the liver, that mass will still be made up of colon cancer cells and the patient will be treated for metastatic colon cancer, not liver cancer. See Question 1 for more information.

2. Only old people get cancer

Statistically, the risk of cancer goes up with age. But although cancer is rare in children and young adults, it is one of the leading causes of death by disease for that age group. In fact, the incidence of some cancers, like colorectal, breast, and prostate, is increasing in adults under the age of fifty. The rising rates of early-onset cancers are a concern because many people in this age group are too young for the recommended screenings. This means their cancer could go undetected for much longer before it is found. See Question 2 and Question 19 for more information.

3. There are "superfoods" or special supplements that can prevent or even cure cancer

Although many supplements are promoted as alternative cancer treatments, there is no evidence that they are effective, and some may have unexpected side effects. "Superfoods" may offer antioxidants and other benefits, but they cannot prevent or cure cancer alone. Stronger evidence supports maintaining a healthy diet and lifestyle to lower cancer risk. Certain foods and supplements may complement conventional cancer therapy, especially if they help with symptoms and side effects, but they must be used carefully to avoid harmful interactions. Just because something is touted as natural does not automatically imply it is safe. To learn more, see Question 40.

4. Living near power lines causes cancer

Other misconceptions about cancer causes include cell phone use, antiperspirants, and artificial sweeteners. However, studies have not shown a clear link between these and cancer. At best, the evidence is inconclusive. Although some lifestyle or environmental factors can be classed as probable or possible carcinogens, it is far more constructive to focus on well-established and preventable risks, such as tobacco use, obesity, and sunburn. See Question 12 and Question 18 for more information.

5. People with dark or tanned skin do not get skin cancer

Anyone with skin can get skin cancer. Darker skin may make it statistically less likely, but it is still a risk. The extra melanin in tanned or darker skin only provides a sun protection factor (SPF) of about 2 to 10. A suntan is still sun-damaged skin, and it could still cause skin cancer down the road. This is significant because people who believe they are protected from skin cancer may neglect sun protection or overlook early warning signs. This topic is discussed in greater detail in Question 16 and Question 17.

Questions and Answers

Cancer Basics

1. What is cancer?

Cancer is a disease of the cells. It occurs when cells grow and spread uncontrollably. This breakdown of normal cell behavior is triggered by genetic errors which cause cells to ignore or subvert their programming. It can occur in almost any kind of tissue, almost anywhere in the body. It is not a new disease, it has existed as long as living organisms have had cells. By understanding how and why cancer develops, scientists and doctors can work toward better ways to prevent, detect, and treat it.

The word cancer is a generic term which refers to over 200 distinct types and subtypes of the disease. This is because there are over 200 different types of cells in the human body, and each of these has the potential to mutate and develop its own specific cancer. Cancers are usually designated by where they first appear. For example, pancreatic cancer is a disease of the cells of the pancreas. It is distinct from colon cancer which is a disease of the cells in the colon. These two cancers will appear and act differently, and they will therefore receive different treatment. Cancers are named and divided into several types based on the kinds of tissues and organs that are affected, and, more frequently nowadays, they are also categorized by their unique molecular features.

Normally, healthy cells grow and divide to replace old or damaged cells, keeping your body in balance. Cancer cells disrupt this balance when these cells do not die off and, instead, begin to multiply without stopping. The corrupted cells stop being part of the collective and start to compete (and outcompete) normal cells for space and resources. A tumor, which is an abnormal and uncontrolled collection of rapidly multiplying cells, can be benign (non-cancerous) or malignant (cancerous). Tumors can recruit their own blood supply which feeds their continued growth.

A malignant tumor's cells can break off from their point of origin and travel to other parts of the body in a process called metastasis, eventually invading other organs and tissues. The more cancer spreads, the harder it is to treat, which makes it a particularly insidious and relentless disease. Some cancers are slow growing, some are aggressive, some are easy to find and easy to treat, some are hidden and deadly.

Cancer has many causes and some of them are still poorly understood. The genetic errors that change healthy cells into cancer can occur for many reasons, but in most cases, they happen simply by chance during cell division. There are, however, many known risk factors which can increase the chance of developing cancer. These factors are based on age, family history, health conditions, environmental exposure, and lifestyle. Sometimes a genetic mutation that increases the risk of getting cancer can be inherited from your parents. Cancer can be associated with multiple, overlapping risk factors, and because it can take several mutations and many years for cancer to develop into a tumor, it is often difficult to pinpoint exact causes.

Although no cancer is entirely preventable, some cancers are considered potentially preventable because their risk factors can be reduced or controlled. The ways of lowering the risk of cancer include diet and exercise, limiting exposure to carcinogens, getting certain vaccines, and following screening guidelines to make early detection more likely. Cancer prevention measures can not only help avoid the disease, but also the burden it imposes on health, finances, relationships, and lifestyle. Unfortunately, cancer is unpredictable. You should never assume that it cannot happen. It can appear in people who seem to have no risk factors, whereas some people at elevated risk might never develop it at all.

A cancer diagnosis can be both shocking and overwhelming. An evaluation will often include a physical exam, imaging, laboratory tests, and a biopsy, where cell samples are examined microscopically. Sometimes genetic testing is done. This can help predict which treatment will be most effective. Once the type of cancer is determined, the doctor or medical team will be able to narrow down the appropriate treatment based on all the information collected.

The most common treatments for cancer are surgery, chemotherapy, and radiation. Cancer treatments have the reputation of being nearly as lethal as the disease they are meant to treat. But new therapies being developed are targeting certain cancers more precisely, reducing the collateral damage to healthy tissue. Still, the effectiveness of cancer treatments must be weighed against their side effects. Some therapies are curative, meaning they eliminate the cancer altogether. Some therapies manage the disease, meaning they can help control or suppress cancer progression, or prevent cancer from recurring. This way, even metastatic cancer can sometimes be treated like a chronic disease.

The field of oncology, the study and treatment of cancer, has been rapidly advancing in recent years due to major breakthroughs in cancer biology. Precision, or personalized, medicine, a medical model that is based on the patient's unique genetic information, is playing an increasingly important role in new cancer treatments. Advances in imaging are improving the chances of early detection, and experts are even seeing how artificial intelligence might be able to improve diagnostic and therapeutic approaches.

Given the prevalence of cancer, the importance of understanding it is critical. Everyone should be empowered to learn about risks and be proactive about prevention. Cancer is not a disease that can be eradicated, but it could be a disease that we can prevent or easily survive.

2. How common is cancer?

Cancer is common, and almost everyone will be affected by the disease at some point, either by getting it or knowing someone who has it. Cancer is the second leading cause of death in the world. According to the World Health Organization (WHO), 1 in 5 people worldwide will be diagnosed with cancer in their lifetime, and 1 in 9 men and 1 in 12 women will die of the disease.

Global cancer rates are difficult to assess because not all countries collect and report their data in the same way. But based on the latest reports, cancer incidence (new cases) and mortality rates (deaths per 100,000) are on the rise worldwide. According to figures released by the International Agency for Research on Cancer (IARC), there were nearly 20 million new cancer cases and 9.7 million cancer deaths in 2022. They predict that by 2050, new cancer cases will increase by 77 percent, and cancer deaths will reach 18.5 million worldwide.

This report, published in 2024, covers 185 countries and thirty-six types of cancer. The most commonly occurring cancers, not including non-melanoma skin cancers, are lung, breast, colorectal, prostate, and stomach. Lung cancer is the leading cause of cancer death, followed by colorectal, liver, breast, and stomach cancer. Worldwide, breast cancer is the most common cancer diagnosed in women, and the most common cause of death. For men, lung cancer is the most common cancer diagnosis and the most common cause of death. Richer countries tend to show high numbers of new cases and lower numbers of deaths, because screening is more advanced, and care is more accessible. In poorer countries, the higher death rate relative to new cases reflects the fact that people are diagnosed later and have less access to care.

In the United States, cancer is the second leading cause of death behind heart disease, and together they make up nearly half of all deaths. One out of every five deaths is due to cancer. According to the Centers for Disease Control and Prevention (CDC), in 2020, the latest year for which there is available data, 1.6 million new cases were reported, and over 602,000 people died of cancer. For every 100,000 people, 403 were newly diagnosed and 144 died. The American Cancer Society (ACS) is expecting 2024 to be the first year that new cancer cases top the 2 million mark, and they project over 611,000 cancer deaths.

According to the National Cancer Institute (NCI), one in two men and one in three women in the United States will be diagnosed with cancer during their lifetime. Men are also more likely than women to die from the disease. Among all demographic groups, non-Hispanic Black men and non-Hispanic white women have the highest rates of new cancer diagnoses. Cancer-related deaths are most common among non-Hispanic Black men, while non-Hispanic Asian/Pacific Islander women experience the lowest mortality rates.

In terms of specific types, prostate cancer is the most frequently diagnosed cancer in men, while breast cancer is the most frequently diagnosed cancer in women. However, lung cancer remains the leading cause of cancer death for both sexes. As of 2024, the ten most common cancer diagnoses in the United States were projected to be breast, prostate, lung and bronchus, colorectal, melanoma, bladder, kidney, non-Hodgkin lymphoma, uterine, and pancreatic cancer.

According to the American Childhood Cancer Organization (ACCO), approximately 1 in 285 children will be diagnosed with cancer before their twentieth birthday. For children in the United States, cancer is the most common cause of death by disease. Nevertheless, childhood cancer is very rare. The most common types of cancer in children are leukemia, lymphoma, brain tumors, and other central nervous system tumors. Cancer in children is often the result of genetic changes that take place during fetal development and is not as strongly linked to lifestyle or environmental risks. This is why children tend to have rarer types of cancer.

Although the number of United States cancer deaths is on the rise, life expectancy has also risen. Cancer is a disease that becomes more common as we age, and it is one of the prices we pay for longevity. When the figures are age-standardized to take life expectancy into account, statistics show that the cancer mortality rate has dropped by 34 percent from 1991 to 2022. This drop is due in part because of a general reduction in smoking, better and earlier detection, and improved treatments. These are also the reasons why five-year survival rates are improving.

And yet, new cases are still on the rise. This is partly the effect of better screening, which finds more cancers earlier, and an aging population that is living longer than before. We are seeing more cancer cases because we are getting better at finding cancer. But the rise in new cases is also due to an increase in other risk factors such as obesity and sedentary lifestyles. There is progress in the fight against cancer, but it is not yet keeping pace with the disease.

Cancer mortality rates may be declining in the United States along with traditional risk factors like tobacco and alcohol, but alarming trends show a demographic shift in cancer incidence. There has been a marked rise in early-onset cancers, which are cancers diagnosed in people under the age of fifty. These cancers include four screenable cancers, some of which are even considered preventable: breast, prostate, colorectal, and cervical, according to the ACS. Compared to a decade ago, nearly twice the number of adults under fifty-five are being diagnosed with colorectal cancer. Statistics indicate that women are being diagnosed with breast cancer at younger ages. Incidence of liver cancer is also increasing in women, and there has been a rise in oral cancers associated with human papillomavirus (HPV) infections.

Are there more cancers in young people, or is cancer being found earlier? A rise in incidence tends to mean both, but the fact that these early-onset cancers seem to be particularly aggressive is a troubling public health issue. In some of these cases, young people are not old enough for the recommended screening guidelines. And young people may delay diagnosis because they are unaware of what their symptoms represent, or they believe they are too young to be concerned about cancer. The result is that their cancer goes undetected for much longer.

The early-onset cancer trend is so far unexplained, and more data is needed to react to it, but many of these early-onset cancers are associated with increased rates of obesity. They are likely a combination of multiple factors, some of which could include artificial light exposure, sleep disruption, antibiotic use, ultra-processed foods, and the gut microbiome. Earlier screening and increased awareness are needed, both among young people and their medical providers.

It is important, when looking at statistics, to understand they rarely directly apply to individuals. Trends and scope are much more relevant for researchers, medical professionals, and policy makers. Cancer statistics should also be understood with an awareness of their limits. Statistics concerning incidence and mortality are usually two to four years behind, because of the time required to collect, compile, and analyze the figures. They also rarely include non-melanoma skin cancers because of their high prevalence and low mortality rates.

They are easily treatable, and cancer registries are not required to track them. Most current statistics and projections are based on the years leading up to and through 2020, but it may take a long time before researchers can factor in the full effect of the Covid-19 pandemic.

Given the current cancer trends, how can you put your risk of getting cancer into perspective? A general understanding of the disease is a good start, and knowing what risk actually means is even more important. Absolute risk is the probability of developing cancer over a certain period of time, like a lifetime risk. A man's lifetime risk of developing lung cancer, for example, is 6 percent. So, 6 out of every 100 men will develop lung cancer over the course of their lives.

Relative risk is a ratio between two groups. So, for example, a smoker is twenty-five times more likely to develop cancer than a non-smoker. As a percentage, the relative risk of cancer is 2500 percent higher in smokers than nonsmokers. Understanding what risk means is important because some statistics play better in the headlines than others. It is also important, ultimately, to know that individual risk is really based on a large variety of factors which vary from person to person. (See Question 19—What demographic groups have the highest risk of developing cancer? and Question 20—What is the economic burden of cancer?)

3. How does cancer develop?

Normal cells develop into cancer cells because a genetic mutation has occurred. Mutations, which are changes in the genes, can cause cells to ignore normal cellular behavior, such as how they grow and divide. In essence, the cell's programing has been corrupted. These distortions of normal function cause the cells to multiply uncontrollably until they accumulate into a mass called a tumor. This mass of abnormal cells hides from the immune system and grows until it threatens the tissue around it. It can begin to feed itself by creating its own blood supply, and it can invade other parts of the body. Carcinogenesis, oncogenesis, tumorigenesis, and neoplasia are words that are used to describe the process by which normal cells develop into cancer.

In a multicellular organism, there are tightly controlled cellular behaviors, or pathways, which allow cells to specialize and in turn allow the organism to thrive. This cooperation relies on behaviors that benefit the collective organism. But cells can sometimes mutate and lose this drive to cooperate. They revert to a cellular programming that makes them compete with (and outcompete) normal cells for space and resources at the expense of the collective. Under normal circumstances, if a cell stops behaving normally, the body triggers its death, and the genetic error that caused its abnormal behavior does not get passed on to the next generation of cells. But if a cell with corrupted genes is neither destroyed nor repaired, the damage and the mutations accumulate. Ultimately, these mutations upset the tightly controlled cellular processes and equilibrium which are characteristic of a healthy organism.

Carcinogenesis is the process by which healthy cells gradually become cancer cells. It is a complex series of steps involving many changes at the genetic level. These changes can happen over many years, and scientists are still working to fully understand their causes. The most widely accepted explanation is the multistep model, a framework which outlines three main stages of cancer development: initiation, promotion, and progression.

Initiation is the first critical step. During initiation, a first mutation occurs in a driver gene, which is a gene that controls cellular growth. This permanent genetic change is now passed on to all future generations of that cell. All of these cells will be at higher risk of eventually developing into cancer. Some genetic mutations involved in cancer are inherited, but most are acquired over many years. These changes can happen spontaneously, or be caused by health conditions, lifestyle factors, or through exposure to substances that damage genes.

Promotion is the step during which the mutated cell is encouraged to multiply. Certain substances or conditions, known as promoters, stimulate the abnormal cell to divide and grow. These promoters do not directly cause mutations themselves, but they interact with the functions of the cell to accelerate growth. Estrogen is an example of a tumor promoter, in that by itself it does not initiate a mutation, but it can drive the growth of a mutated cell. Other promoters might include chronic inflammation, certain medications, or chemical exposure. Promotion leads to clonal expansion, where a single mutated cell multiplies into a growing mass of abnormal cells.

Progression is the final step, during which each generation of cells results in unique combinations of genetic features. As the abnormal cells continue dividing, their genes become more unstable, and new mutations appear. The result is a population of cells that all behave differently—some grow faster, some spread more easily, and some become more resistant to the body's defenses. This stage is marked by increased diversity within the tumor, known as heterogeneity. Over time, the cells evolve into a malignant tumor, capable of invading other tissues and spreading throughout the body.

These steps highlight the importance of prevention and early intervention because as cancer becomes more complex, it becomes harder to treat. The multistep model is based on the Somatic Mutation Theory, which states that cancer originates from a single cell's genetic mutation. It is a framework that can explain most cancers, but not all. Some alternative theories of cancer development point to other biological processes, including cellular communication, and chromosomal instability.

The Tissue Organization Field Theory suggests that cancer arises from disruptions in the communication and organization of cells within tissues rather than from genetic mutations. Another model, the Chromosomal Instability Theory, proposes that cancer is a result of chromosomal abnormalities rather than specific mutations. The Mitochondrial Metabolic Theory describes how disrupted energy production in the cell leads to genetic damage caused by an excess of reactive oxygen species (ROS), a highly reactive molecule that is a byproduct of cellular respiration. The implication is that genetic mutations are a downstream effect rather than the direct cause of cancer development.

Most theories indicate that the more cells divide, the higher the risk of mutation, leading to the assumption that the more cells there are, the higher the risk of cancer. Peto's Paradox, however, is the surprising observation that large animals like elephants and whales are less prone to developing cancer than smaller animals, like humans or mice. Large animals have more cells and live longer, so, statistically the risk should increase, but it does not. This suggests that these animals may have evolved some kind of protection against cancer. This paradox, and other alternative models that challenge our assumptions about cancer development, could inspire various new directions of research, potentially leading to better prevention strategies or even a cure. (See Question 4—What role does mutation play in cancer development? and Question 5—What are the hallmarks of cancer?)

4. What role does mutation play in cancer development?

Cancer is a disease of the cells, but it originates in the genes. To track how cancer develops from a normal cell into a malignancy, it is important to understand the mechanisms of normal cell behavior and how it can all go wrong.

How do normal cells behave in the body? There are around 35 trillion cells in the human body, and they are constantly dividing, multiplying, and dying.

Cell division enables our body's growth, development, and repair. When a cell receives the signal to divide, it responds by growing, producing the proteins it needs, duplicating its genes, and finally splitting itself into two new cells through a process called mitosis. This is the normal cycle of a cell.

During the cycle there are checkpoints, quality control mechanisms, which preserve the integrity and stability of cell replication. These checkpoints verify that the sequence of genes is intact and complete. If errors are detected the cell will either repair the damage, or it will trigger a self-destruct sequence. This is called programmed cell death or apoptosis.

This process is crucial because, given the trillions of cells in the human body, and the tens of thousands of genes in the human genome, division errors are statistically inevitable. Under normal circumstances, however, 99 percent of these errors are repaired or eliminated.

Programmed cell death is also important in maintaining regular cell turnover. A cell replicates itself from one cell to two, from two to four, from four to eight and so on. This self-destruct mechanism prunes out old and damaged cells, helping to maintain the required number of cells in the body. The processes of cell division and cell death are tightly controlled.

These mechanisms are all directed by our DNA, which is a molecular copy of the body's manual, the set of instructions, or blueprints. DNA, which stands for deoxyribonucleic acid, is a molecule located in the nucleus of every cell. It is made up of four nucleotide bases: adenine, thymine, guanine, and cytosine. These nucleotides line up in pairs and form a ladder-like structure which is twisted into DNA's characteristic double helix shape. The specific order of the nucleotides is what encodes genetic information. There are 3.2 billion base pairs, and all of them are duplicated every time a cell divides. If DNA is an instruction manual, chromosomes are the chapters, genes are the paragraphs, and nucleotides make up the words.

A chromosome is a long packet of DNA that contains a carefully organized selection of genes. The human genome, the complete set of human DNA, is written into twenty-three pairs of chromosomes. Half of each pair is inherited from the mother, the other half from the father. These will contain mostly the same genes in the same location, as well as mutations inherited from each parent. They will also contain mutations that have occurred during the body's development, all of which come together to make each individual unique. A set of chromosomes is present in the nucleus of almost every cell in the body. When a cell divides, each chromosome is copied and tightly raveled before splitting itself in half.

DNA contains all the instructions for what a cell might do, but genes determine which of these things the cell will do, and how. Genes are linear sequences of nucleotides which, when decoded, provide specific instructions to the cell. They encode an individual's physical traits and directions for cellular activity. All the cells in the body contain the same DNA. But in each cell, certain genes are either expressed (switched on) or repressed (switched off), differentiating the cells, causing them to produce different proteins, making some behave like bone cells and others like muscle cells, and so on.

Genes contain the code to make proteins, which are complex molecules made of amino acids. Proteins regulate cell functions, provide structure, and transport materials and information within the body. When a gene is transcribed, its instructions are copied into a molecule of ribonucleic acid (RNA) inside the cell's nucleus. The RNA acts as a template carrying the genetic instructions out of the nucleus to a structure called the ribosome. The ribosome decodes or translates the RNA instructions and synthesizes the protein by linking amino acids together, according to the original DNA instructions.

When something happens to change the instructions, however, the wrong gene might be switched on or switched off, and the wrong protein, or no protein at all, might be synthesized. These changes in the genes are called mutations. A mutation is a permanent change in DNA structure, an alteration in the nucleotide sequence of the DNA. It is as if somewhere in the instruction manual, certain words or whole paragraphs had been added, moved around, or deleted altogether.

When a mutation occurs, it acts like a typo or an error in the code, and the gene begins to issue faulty instructions. Mutations can instruct the amino acids to form proteins that are inappropriate or ineffective. Sometimes, mutations happen in sections of DNA that are responsible for activating or deactivating other genes. Cells acquire mutations all the time, but not all of them result in cancer and many of them are harmless. Mutations are essential in the process of evolution and adaptation because they generate genetic variation.

Mutations fall into two main categories: germline and somatic. Germline mutations occur in reproductive cells and can be passed down from parent to child, making them hereditary. Somatic mutations arise in nonreproductive cells. While they can be transmitted to dividing cells during mitosis, they are not passed down from parent to child, and are considered acquired.

Some mutations affect just one gene, while others impact the structure of entire chromosomes. Point mutations are changes in a single nucleotide, which might be substituted for another nucleotide, inserted where it does not belong, or simply deleted. Chromosomal mutations involve larger DNA segments and can result in being deleted or duplicated. The chromosomes might also become inverted or moved altogether to another chromosome.

Besides DNA mutations, epigenetic changes also affect gene activity. They can modify the way the genes are expressed, whether they are switched on or off. They come about through environmental or lifestyle factors and can be passed from parent to child. Because they have affected how the cells read the DNA sequence, but not altered the sequence itself, it is possible to reverse epigenetic changes.

Cancer cells come from normal cells, so they carry all the instructions for normal cell behavior. But they corrupt and exploit these instructions, which is why they are so successful at surviving and spreading. So, paradoxically, cancer can turn the systems put in place to stop it to its own advantage. This disruption and undermining of normal cell division is called cell cycle dysregulation.

Normal cells need to multiply for growth, healing, and cellular turnover. Immune cells need to be able to infiltrate and move around the body to address trauma or infection. These cellular functions are critical to life and are tightly controlled. Cancer cells still have this programming, but their specific mutations allow them to operate outside the body's normal control mechanisms. They get around all the safeguards and exploit their ability to multiply abnormally, survive, infiltrate, and spread. And as a result, the cancer cells' defective genes survive generation after generation.

Cancer-causing mutations tend to happen in specific genes. The two main types of genes involved in cancer development are oncogenes and tumor suppressor genes.

The genes responsible for normal cell growth are called proto-oncogenes. Their purpose in the cell is to initiate division, drive activity, and ensure survival. Proto-oncogenes are often compared to a car's accelerator. They drive cellular growth. In cancer development, proto-oncogenes experience gain-of-function mutations, which are mutations that result in new, abnormally increased, or enhanced function. With these mutations they become oncogenes, genes that have cancer-causing potential. With the gain-of-function mutation, they are locked into a state of continuously promoting growth, regardless of the needs of the cell, a process called constitutive activation. Oncogenes are what happens when the accelerator is stuck at full speed.

Tumor suppressor genes are gatekeeper genes that slow or stop cell division when damaged DNA is detected during one of the cell cycle's checkpoints. These genes encode the proteins needed for cell arrest, which is a pause in the cycle.

Cell arrest gives DNA repair genes time to ensure there is a faithful and stable copy of the DNA. DNA repair genes are caretakers that correct the mutations by reverting to the original sequence. Tumor suppressor genes can also trigger programmed cell death or apoptosis. This pausing or stopping of the cycle is crucial in allowing a cell with damaged DNA to be repaired or eliminated.

Tumor suppressor genes are often compared to a car's brakes, they slow or stop a damaged cell before it multiplies. These genes experience loss-of-function mutations, or mutations that result in reduced or terminated function. When they stop functioning, there is no pausing or stopping the cycle, regardless of the genetic damage. A mutation in DNA repair genes causes the unlimited acquisition of more mutations. Mutations survive and multiply. With no cell death, growth is unrestrained. When tumor suppressor genes mutate, the car brakes fail.

Cancer essentially begins with the increased activity of oncogenes and the inactivation of tumor suppressor genes. With a stuck accelerator and failing brakes, a car speeds out of control. For a cell, this loss of control results in excessive and inappropriate proliferation. This is what drives cancer's aggressive growth.

Another way cancer cells cheat cellular death is by becoming immortal. The tip of each chromosome has a specific, repetitive sequence of nucleotides called a telomere. It functions like a cap, or the tip of a shoelace, which protects the chromosome from becoming unraveled or degraded over time. Every time the cell replicates and the chromosome divides, its telomeres become shorter. When the telomere becomes so short the chromosome can no longer be faithfully divided, the cell undergoes a state of cellular aging in which it can no longer replicate, and it eventually dies.

Telomerase is an enzyme that maintains and rebuilds the telomere. It is active in sperm and egg cells where it maintains the integrity of the DNA that is passed on to the next generation. This activity is reduced or switched off in normal cells after birth so the telomeres can do their job of stopping cells from dividing with frayed chromosomes. However, some cancer cells develop a mutation that reactivates telomerase. This mutation prevents cellular aging and essentially makes the cancer cells immortal. They will replicate forever but never die.

Generally, cancer is monoclonal, meaning the disease originates with a mutation in a single abnormal cell. But carcinogenesis is not the result of just one event. It is the result of an accumulation of mutations. An initial mutation might make a cell capable of dividing faster. Its daughter cells would inherit this mutation and eventually develop another. Depending on the type, cancer is the result of three to twenty different mutations that have occurred progressively, sometimes over many years. The lineage from that single mutated cell will deviate, over time, moving further and further from the behavior and appearance of normal cells.

Cells naturally mutate at a very low rate, with about one mutation in every 100 million cell generations. But each mutation makes a subsequent one more likely. In cancer cells, mutations happen at a much higher rate, about once every 1000 cell generations. So, each error in DNA replication results in more and more subsequent errors. This is why cancers are most likely to develop in cells that divide very frequently.

5. What are the hallmarks of cancer?

Cancer development is not consistent, it varies depending on cancer type and location. It is not always caused by the same set of mutations in the same order. It is a complex and adaptive process. But scientists have determined that all cancer cells do have certain features in common. In 2000, Bob Weinberg and Douglas Hanahan published a paper called "Hallmarks of Cancer" which collected the key elements that apply to all cancers. They have since followed up with two more emerging hallmarks and two enabling characteristics as research into cancer's molecular makeup has progressed. Cancer cells possess the following hallmarks:

1. Sustained proliferative signaling—Normal cells only divide when they receive a growth signal. But the oncogenes that trigger cellular division and growth are now constantly activated and cancer cells are driven to divide even without such a signal. The cells begin to work independently to stimulate their own growth.
2. Evading growth suppressors—Mutations switch off tumor suppressor genes, so cancer cells can ignore signals to stop dividing. This makes it harder to repair or eliminate genetic damage.
3. Resisting cell death—Mutations that deactivate the genes that control cell death allow cancer cells to escape destruction. Cancer cells avoid normal turnover and begin to accumulate more and more genetic damage because they do not know when to die.
4. Enabling replicative immortality—Telomeres, the protective caps at the ends of chromosomes, are continually lengthened, which prevents

the natural onset of cell cycle arrest and cell death. This allows for infinite generations of daughter cells.

5. Inducing angiogenesis—Angiogenesis is the growth of new blood vessels. Certain tumor cells harness the ability to bring in capillaries from nearby blood vessels. These provide a source of nutrients, oxygen, and waste removal. Access to the circulatory system also allows cancer cells to spread out into the body.
6. Activating invasion and metastasis—Normal cells stop growing when they encounter other cells, and for the most part, they do not travel around the body. Cancer cells ignore normal cellular constraints and crowd out and invade surrounding tissues. They can also travel throughout the body through the circulatory or lymphatic system.

Two emerging hallmarks and two enabling characteristics were added to this list in 2011.

7. Deregulating cellular energetics—The metabolism of cancer cells changes as they develop alternative ways to make energy. These pathways, though inefficient, allow them to build more cells and can also help them adapt to what would otherwise be hostile conditions in the body.
8. Avoiding immune destruction—Whereas damaged or abnormal cells are usually eliminated by the immune system, cancer cells escape destruction by hiding from or disabling the immune response.

These hallmarks are made possible by two enabling characteristics:

Genome instability and mutation—The accumulation and excessive number of mutations result in extreme changes in the number and "architecture" of the chromosomes. Some cancer cells have many more than the normal number of chromosomes. And because each mutation makes the next one more likely, the genomic abnormalities in cancer cells increase and worsen as the disease progresses.

Tumor-promoting inflammation—Inflammation is the immune system's response to damage. It attacks infection and stimulates tissue repair. However, cancer cells can initiate and exploit an inflammatory response from the immune system by using the growth factors produced by immune cells to grow more cancer cells. They can also trick the immune system into protecting the tumor rather than attacking it.

The hallmarks are fundamental changes in cancer cells, acquired through mutations, which allow them to multiply and spread. They provide a unifying framework and a foundation for research even though cancers differ in so many complex ways. Understanding the hallmarks of cancer can help target therapies and improve diagnosis and prevention strategies.

6. What is a tumor?

The term "tumor" is broadly used for masses, swellings, or cysts, but in the context of cancer, it refers to a lump or growth made up of abnormal cells. A tumor, which is more accurately called a neoplasm ("neo" meaning new, and "plasma" meaning formation), happens when an overgrowth of cells has accumulated into a mass of new tissue. This process is called tumorigenesis, or neoplasia. Not all tumors are cancer, but they are a sign of cellular dysfunction. Tumors can be painful but sometimes cause no symptoms or discomfort at all.

Tumors form because their cells no longer behave like normal cells. When normal cells divide and proliferate, they begin to crowd and touch each other. As this happens, they slow down their rate of division. This is a process called contact inhibition. A cut in the skin will heal by creating new cells. When the wound surface has filled in, contact inhibition shuts down production. It keeps the number of cells in balance during tissue regrowth. Mutated cells, however, are being driven to multiply uncontrollably. They lose contact inhibition and keep dividing and amassing even though they are in contact with neighboring cells. They overflow the space they would normally be restricted to and start forming a mass.

Various terms describe a tumor's tissue changes based on the appearance of its cells. Hypertrophy is an increase in the size of the cells. Hyperplasia is an increase in the number of cells, even though they still appear normal. At this point, these changes are normal adaptive and healing behaviors, the cells' genes are still normal, and the change is reversible.

Cells that are referred to as having atypia are beginning to appear abnormal or damaged. Metaplasia describes the process whereby one type of cell is replaced with another type of cell that is not typically found in that tissue. Dysplasia is characterized by abnormal growth, and a disorganized structure. These changes are generally the result of a specific stimulus, like an infection and can sometimes be reversible.

Neoplasia is the term that describes tissue changes which are considered irreversible. The tissue is referred to as autonomous because it no longer depends on outside signals to change. As it grows and becomes more disorganized, it becomes more prone to developing into cancer. Sometimes the cells of a tumor become dedifferentiated, meaning they are reverting to a less developed, less specialized form. They are referred to as anaplastic, meaning "formed backward." They are becoming more like stem cells and therefore better able to self-renew, adapt, and spread. Anaplastic cells grow aggressively and tend to resist treatment.

Cells inside a tumor are the product of generations of progressive and random mutations. These generations develop different variants, and the tumor becomes more heterogeneous, meaning it consists of many different kinds of cells. As the tumor develops, its mutation-prone cells become increasingly adaptable. This results in a mass that can change quickly, making it harder for the immune system to find and fight, and easier for it to evade treatment.

Tumor heterogeneity is one of the biggest challenges in treating cancer because not all cells within the same tumor will respond to therapy the same way. This can lead to drug resistance and recurrence. In a way, cancer is not really one single disease, even within the same tumor.

Not all cancers develop into solid tumors. Liquid tumors refer to cancer cells that circulate through the bloodstream or lymphatic system. Cells in liquid tumors undergo similar stages of change and are similarly characterized by abnormal proliferation, although they move throughout a system and are not stuck in a single location.

There are three kinds of tumors: benign, premalignant, and malignant. These are distinguished by their degree of invasiveness, or potential to spread around the body.

Benign tumors are noncancerous. They are generally slow growing and often well differentiated, which means the cells look normal and organized. They are usually encapsulated, meaning they have a distinct border layer and are clearly discrete or separate from the surrounding tissue. The reason they are localized is that, although they may increase in size, they are constrained by the surrounding tissue and unable to move into other tissue or split off into another part of the body.

Tumors are always monitored because they are essentially an abnormal development, and though unlikely, some benign tumors could turn into cancer. A benign tumor does not always cause symptoms, and in many cases, doctors will simply monitor it. But depending on where it is located, it can cause disfigurement, discomfort, or pain. Although it is not cancer, if it grows large enough to restrict blood flow, or compress nearby organs or nerves, it can present a serious health risk or even be fatal. The solution is usually surgical removal, sometimes medication, and very occasionally radiation. Because benign tumors are localized and well defined, they are not prone to growing back once they are removed.

Premalignant, or precancerous tumors, are different from benign tumors in that they have the potential for developing into cancer. They are genetically unstable, and it may be a matter of time before they progress into cancer. Premalignant tumor cells vary in appearance from normal to disorganized with invasive potential. These tumors are also sometimes called preinvasive.

Some noninvasive cancers are considered premalignant. Carcinoma in situ (CIS) is considered premalignant, or pre-cancer, because it has not invaded the supporting structure in which it is growing. "In situ" means "in its place," and although these tumors' cells look the same as invasive cancer cells, they are not yet capable of spreading. It is impossible to predict whether premalignant tumors will become malignant if left untreated, but the risk can be significant, so they are usually treated and removed if possible.

Malignant tumors are masses that are about to, or have already become, invasive. They are cancer. This ability to invade is what differentiates cancer from any other mass of abnormal cells. Malignant tumors are often aggressive. They are undifferentiated, or poorly differentiated, meaning the cells look immature and disorganized compared to healthy cells nearby. They will push against surrounding cells and become embedded into the surrounding or basement membrane. They may grow new blood vessels. They now have the potential to spread to other parts of the body, extending to other organs nearby or breaking off into the bloodstream. As malignant tumors expand and grow, their functions become more complex. This makes them harder to treat and more likely to reappear after treatment.

Cancer names reflect their tumors' cellular origin and behavior. They are named by pairing the name of the affected body part or tissue with the suffix "oma," which is a Greek root meaning swelling. This suffix applies to both benign and malignant tumors. So, an adenoma ("adeno"—gland and "oma"—tumor) is a benign tumor in glandular tissue. The term "adenocarcinoma" ("adeno"—gland, "carcin"—cancer, and "oma"—tumor) implies the tumor is malignant.

A tumor, which is a dynamic and evolving tissue, exists in the body in its own ecosystem called the tumor microenvironment. Tumors are not isolated, they interact with their surroundings, manipulating nearby cells to help them grow and survive. The tumor microenvironment includes immune cells, blood vessels, and connective tissue. It is all supported in a molecular scaffold, a structure called the extracellular matrix, which holds everything together.

As a tumor grows, it changes the microenvironment to suit its needs. Like healthy tissue, tumors require oxygen, nutrients, and the removal of metabolic waste. A very small tumor can do this through a process called passive diffusion, in which molecules simply move back and forth across the cell membrane.

But when a tumor grows beyond a certain size (1–3 mm in diameter), it can no longer support its microenvironment. The tumor cells begin to suffer from hypoxia, or oxygen deficiency, which stimulates the growth of new blood vessels in a process called angiogenesis. Although angiogenesis is a normal function in growth and wound healing, tumors often harness this process to grow.

Angiogenesis is a common feature of the tumor microenvironment. It is associated with increasing the tumor's aggressiveness and resistance to therapies. Because the new vessels formed in the tumor are made of dysfunctional cancer cells, they are disorganized and leaky, which helps them penetrate the bloodstream and spread. It also reduces the effectiveness of getting cancer treating drugs into the tumor through the bloodstream.

Tumors can hijack immune responses and use inflammation to fuel growth or hide from immune system attacks. This means the body might unintentionally protect the tumor instead of fighting it. How a tumor progresses and changes is a result of how it interacts with its microenvironment, which evolves as the tumor develops. The tumor microenvironment adds another layer of complexity to the treatment of cancer. (See Question 35—How does immunotherapy work, and what are the potential side effects?)

Cancer cells tend to grow faster than the tumor's inefficient blood vessels can nourish them. So, another key feature of the tumor microenvironment is the abnormal way cancer cells make energy. Normal cells use a process called cellular respiration, in which the mitochondria (which are the powerhouse of the cell) break down nutrients to produce energy. Unlike normal cells, many cancer cells rely on aerobic glycolysis, which is a process of quickly breaking down glucose or sugars, without oxygen, even when oxygen is present. One explanation for this is that damage to the mitochondrial DNA interferes with cellular respiration and forces the cells to produce energy differently.

This phenomenon, known as the Warburg effect, is less efficient and yields less energy. But like many of cancer's crude distortions of normal cellular behavior, this kind of energy production does offer some benefits to the tumor. Aerobic glycolysis produces lactic acid, making the environment more acidic. This acidity can suppress the immune system, which normally destroys abnormal cells, and helps cancer cells survive and grow.

Aerobic glycolysis also produces a variety of byproducts that the tumor then uses to make more cancer cells. As a result, cancer cells are extremely hungry for glucose, they metabolize twenty times more of it than normal cells. This characteristic is useful for tracking malignancies in the body with positron emission tomography (PET) scanning. During this scan, radioactively tagged glucose lights up where it is concentrated in the glucose-hungry tumor. Understanding more about how and why cancer cells metabolize fuel the way they do could lead to more targets for cancer therapies.

Over time, as the tumor continues to grow and mutate, the microenvironment evolves and adapts with it. These changes can turn the cancer into a more aggressive malignancy, making it harder for the immune system or drugs to stop it. The tumor's ability to fuel the evolution of therapy resistant cancer cell populations is the reason most cancers are treated with multiple therapies. And because of this, scientists are increasingly developing therapies that target not just the tumor, but also the features of its surrounding environment.

7. What is metastasis?

Metastasis is the term used to describe how cancer cells separate from a tumor and spread to other tissues and organs in the body. It is cancer's deadliest trait, and the unquestionable sign that a tumor is malignant. Metastasis is the major cause of mortality in cancer cases because of the damage it causes to vital tissues, and the disruption to essential body functions.

The initial tumor is referred to as the primary tumor. When pieces of it migrate through the body, they form new, or secondary tumors. These new tumor cells will be the same as the original cancer's cells. So, if a cancerous tumor in the colon spreads to the liver, that mass will still be made of colon cancer cells, and the patient will be treated for metastatic colon cancer, not liver cancer. The metastasis will keep the name of the original cancer.

Metastasis is found using screenings, scans, and tests. If the tissue biopsy reveals the cells are the same as the primary cancer, the diagnosis is metastatic cancer. Liquid biopsies, blood tests that can detect circulating tumor cells, are being used increasingly to identify metastatic disease in the body. These tests can reveal metastasis earlier than using imaging and are less invasive than a traditional biopsy.

Sometimes a metastatic tumor is found before the primary cancer. Although the tumor cells might clearly indicate they came from elsewhere in the body, it may be impossible to pinpoint exactly where, in which case the diagnosis will be cancer of unknown primary origin. Nearly all cancers can metastasize. The exceptions are brain cancer and basal cell carcinoma. The damage these two cancers cause is by local invasion, where they grow so large they can restrict circulation and destroy nearby tissue.

There is no medical cure for most metastatic cancers. There are, however, many treatments that can manage or control the disease by stopping or slowing its spread. Widespread disease can be addressed with systemic treatments like chemotherapy or immunotherapy. In these cases, cancer can be managed like a chronic illness, sometimes for years. But metastatic cells are genetically unstable and often become resistant to treatment. If a patient's cancer can no longer be controlled, or if they can no longer tolerate the treatment, they will, at this point, receive palliative care to minimize pain, limit symptoms, and preserve quality of life.

Exactly what initiates the process of metastasis is still unclear. Several factors can trigger it. Metastasis is most likely to occur in tumors where there is aggressive growth or where certain genetic changes have given the cells the potential to spread. Changes in the tumor microenvironment, such as an increase in acidity or a decrease in oxygen, might be a cause. Even cancer treatments like chemotherapy could be a trigger. Killing off some cells in the tumor could cause other surviving cells to become more active and capable of migrating.

The process of metastasis is called the metastatic cascade. It is an ordered series of events that requires specific cellular functions. First, a tumor will extend and separate itself into a clump of cells, move through the membrane and tissue that surrounds it, and penetrate neighboring tissue. This is called local invasion.

The next step is intravasation, during which the cancer cells enter the blood or lymphatic system and circulate. These systems are hostile to cancer cells which are effectively foreign bodies, but these cells adapt quickly and are very good at surviving.

The circulating tumor cells will eventually exit the vessels in a process called extravasation. This happens, sometimes, because the vessels simply end or narrow. Sometimes the cells follow the direction of drainage from the primary tumor to the nearest organ. Sometimes they exit because they have found a welcoming environment that encourages their survival. This process is explained by the seed and soil hypothesis in that the seed will travel until it finds the kind of soil that will help it grow.

If the tumor cells survive the journey, wherever they emerge, they will try to colonize and grow in this secondary site. These are disseminated cancer cells, and they can remain dormant for months or years, either in the circulatory system or at the secondary site. It is impossible to predict where or when these cells will escape tumor dormancy, which is part of why metastasis is such a problem.

A cancer's origin will often dictate where it is likely to spread. Colon cancer tends to metastasize in the liver and lungs, breast cancer tends to metastasize to the bones and brain. The most common sites of metastasis include the lymph nodes, adrenal glands, bones, brain, liver, lungs, and the peritoneum, which is the membrane that lines the abdominal cavity. These sites are vulnerable because they are hubs of fluid circulation or downstream destinations for various circulatory vessels.

The two most common pathways for metastasis are through the lymphatic system and the circulatory system. The lymphatic system is the part of the immune system which manages, moves, and purifies body fluids. Its network reaches every part of the body, which is how cancer cells use it to spread.

Some cancers are hematogenous, meaning they travel in the blood through the circulatory system. They tend to exit the blood vessels and lodge into the first capillary beds they find, which is why the liver and lungs are common sites for metastasis.

The third pathway for metastasis is transcoelomic spread, which occurs when the tumor cells grow directly through membranes into surrounding tissue, or into the abdominal or chest cavities.

Metastasis is what makes cancer such a relentless and deadly disease. According to the National Cancer Institute's (NCI) Surveillance, Epidemiology, and End Results (SEER) program, data from 2012 to 2018 showed that the five-year survival rate for female breast cancer was 99.1 percent if diagnosed while it was still localized. That rate dropped to 30 percent for a diagnosis of metastatic breast cancer. Because of metastasis, the earlier the cancer can be found, the better the outcome for the patient.

8. What are the different types of cancer?

Cancers are classified by primary site or by tissue type. Classifying by primary site means sorting cancers based on where in the body, or in which organ, the cancer first appeared. Classifying by tissue type is sorting cancers by the specific kinds of cells in which the cancer first developed. Medical professionals generally classify cancers by tissue type. This is known as histologic classification because it looks at the microscopic features of the cells. There are as many different kinds of cancers as there are different kinds of cells in the body, which is why this kind of classification is important for making a precise diagnosis and identifying appropriate treatment plans. It is also important for researchers and cancer registries to be able to track the disease using a consistent system.

Recently, there has been a shift toward classifying cancers based on molecular or genetic profiling rather than by site or tissue of origin. Molecular-based classification aligns with advances in precision, or personalized medicine, which uses genetic testing of tumor cells to identify treatment targets. Molecular profiling examines genes and chromosomes as well as proteins, biomarkers, and other molecules that provide a deeper understanding of cancer's behavior. This approach not only improves the accuracy of cancer diagnoses, but also leads to more personalized care, and helps regulatory agencies move more efficiently in approving cancer drugs.

The World Health Organization (WHO) has created a single unified classification system based on malignancy, site of origin, tissue type, grade, spread, and in some cases, molecular features. This is not only an effective tool for diagnosing and determining treatment, but it helps focus policy decisions about research and drug development. It is also increasingly useful for harnessing artificial intelligence in the fight against cancer. The International Classification of Diseases for Oncology, Third Edition (ICD-O-3) developed by the WHO, classifies cancers using six major categories: carcinomas, sarcomas, leukemias, lymphomas, myelomas, and mixed types.

Cancers are divided into two general categories: solid tumor cancers and hematologic, or blood cancers. Solid tumor cancers form a mass or multiple masses in and around organs. Blood cancers, also referred to as liquid tumors, begin in the bone marrow, blood, or lymph nodes, and then travel throughout the circulatory or lymphatic systems. Carcinomas and sarcomas are solid tumor cancers whereas leukemia, lymphoma, and myeloma are blood cancers.

Carcinoma—Carcinoma is the most common type of cancer. The National Cancer Institute (NCI) estimates that it accounts for 80 to 90 percent of all cancers. Carcinoma is cancer of the epithelial cells, which are cells that make up the interior and exterior lining of the body. This includes skin and tissues that line or cover organs, tracts, and ducts. Epithelial tissue is protective, its cells suffer damage often and are healed and renewed constantly. It is this feature which makes mutations more likely to occur there. Carcinoma typically tends to spread and metastasize into lymph nodes, although in the later stages of the disease they will also spread through the blood. There are two main subtypes, adenocarcinomas, and squamous cell carcinomas. These are further classified by the specific epithelial cells they affect.

An adenocarcinoma is a tumor that forms in organs or glands whose cells generate mucus and fluids. These kinds of cells are found in the lining of organs such as the colon, where the cells secrete mucus, or the pancreas where the cells secrete insulin. These types of glandular cells are also present in the breast, lung, and prostate.

Squamous cell carcinoma affects the thin, flat cells in the squamous epithelium, which is directly under the outer surface of the skin. Squamous cells can also line various hollow organs like the stomach, bladder, uterus, or kidney.

Sarcoma—Tumors that develop in supportive or connective tissues are collectively called sarcomas. These tissues include bone, tendon, ligament, cartilage, as well as soft tissue like muscle and fat. Sarcomas mimic the appearance of the tissue in which they are growing. They most often spread through blood vessels because connective tissues have less access to the lymphatic system. Sarcomas are relatively rare and represent a small percentage of cancer diagnoses in adults. They are more common in pediatric cancer cases. Osteosarcoma, a type of bone cancer, and leiomyosarcoma, cancer of the smooth muscle, are the most frequently diagnosed sarcomas.

Leukemia—Leukemia is a blood cancer, and the tenth most common cancer in the United States. It develops in the blood-forming cells of bone marrow, specifically in lymphoblastic or myeloid cells. This cancer causes the body to produce excessive amounts of abnormal white blood cells. These abnormal cells displace normal blood cells and platelets, leading to anemia or low iron. This makes it harder for the body to oxygenate and regulate immune responses like fighting infections. Leukemia can develop into a chronic or acute disease, meaning some forms worsen much faster than others. Acute lymphocytic leukemia is one of the most common forms of leukemia. It mainly affects young children.

Lymphoma—Lymphoma, a relatively rare blood cancer, affects lymphocytes, a type of disease-fighting white blood cell in the lymphatic system. The lymphatic system is the part of the immune system which manages, moves, and purifies body fluids. Lymphomas generally develop in the lymph nodes, where abnormal cells proliferate so much the nodes become enlarged and can no longer function properly. There are two main types of lymphoma, Hodgkin lymphoma and non-Hodgkin lymphoma. Hodgkin lymphoma is less common and is characterized by the presence of a specific kind of abnormal cell, called Reed-Sternberg. It is a treatable and curable form of cancer. Non-Hodgkin lymphomas, classified by which type of white blood cells are affected, are harder to treat. Although lymphoma is a blood cancer, it can sometimes result in the formation of solid masses.

Myeloma—Myeloma is a cancer that originates inside the bone marrow, in plasma cells. Plasma cells are the immune cells that produce antibodies. When these cells become cancerous, they proliferate and grow in the bone marrow of the spine. In the case of multiple myeloma, these cells can travel to other bone marrow and build up throughout the body. It is a very rare cancer. In the United States, the risk of developing multiple myeloma is less than 1 percent.

Mixed types—Mixed type cancers have elements of different cancers, within one type or across many types of cancer. For example, a carcinosarcoma is a tumor that has the microscopic tissue structure of both carcinoma and sarcoma because it is made up of both glandular and squamous cells.

Some other malignancies fall outside these categories. Certain brain and spinal cord tumors occur in neural tissues. Germ cell tumors appear in the cells that develop into reproductive cells, eggs in the ovaries, and sperm in the testes. Blastoma is a cancer of immature or precursor cells, which are called blasts. This type of cancer is more common in children and can occur in various organs around the body. Neuroendocrine carcinomas are rare tumors that form in the specialized cells of the hormone-secreting neuroendocrine system.

9. Where in the body can I get cancer, and which cancers are most common?

Cancer is often categorized by the place in the body where the cancer first appeared, which is called the primary site. Lung cancer is cancer that first appeared in the lung, breast cancer is cancer that first appeared in the breast. This method of categorizing cancers is less accurate but easier to understand than tissue typing or molecular profiling. It is less accurate because there are different types of lung and breast cancers with different molecular profiles, but it is more logical for non-medical people to break down the disease by location first, and tissue type second.

There are over 200 different types and subtypes of cancer, and many of them are very rare. According to the American Cancer Society (ACS), the most common places where cancer occurs are the skin, breast, prostate, lung, colon, and rectum. Roughly ten to twelve types of cancer make up the bulk of all cancer cases worldwide. Breast, lung, colorectal, and prostate cancers account for nearly 50 percent of all new cancer diagnoses in the United States.

Skin Cancer—Skin cancer is the most common type of cancer, developing in the outer layer of the skin called the epidermis. It usually appears in areas that are exposed to sunlight but can also develop in other places like the palms of the hands and soles of the feet, or in the genital area. Skin cancers are generally caused by exposure to the sun's ultraviolet (UV) rays, or artificial sources of radiation such as sun lamps and tanning beds, but a compromised or weakened immune system is also a risk factor. People with pale skin which is prone to freckling and sunburn, or people with a history of serious sunburn, are especially at risk. Squamous and basal cell carcinomas are the most common types of skin cancer.

Squamous cell carcinoma of the skin affects cells in the middle and outer layers of skin, just under the surface. It may appear as a bump or nodule, or a rough scabby sore. Basal cell carcinoma is a cancer that originates in the base layer of the skin, under the squamous cells. Basal cells produce new skin cells which push the older cells to the surface of the skin. This carcinoma often appears as a pink, brown, or black growth, or a sore that does not heal. Squamous and basal cell carcinomas can be dangerous if left untreated as they can grow quite deep, but when caught early, they can often be removed completely. These kinds of cancers are common, often detected early, and treated easily, sometimes in a single visit to a dermatologist. They are therefore not as accurately tracked on national and international cancer registries, which is one of the reasons cancer statistics often exclude nonmelanoma skin cancers.

Melanoma is a form of skin cancer that develops in the melanocytes, which are cells that produce melanin. Melanin is responsible for pigmentation and for protecting the skin from the dangerous effects of UV radiation. Melanocytes are cells located in the basal layers of the skin, and a few other areas around the body like the hair and eyes, and some internal organs. A melanoma will often overproduce melanin, resulting in a deep brown or black lesion on the skin. Melanoma is the most serious kind of skin cancer because it grows aggressively and spreads quickly.

Kaposi sarcoma is a rare cancer that originates in the cells lining the skin, lymph nodes, or mucous membranes, causing tumors or lesions. This cancer is caused by the Kaposi sarcoma-associated herpesvirus (KSHV). Most people who have had this viral infection will never get Kaposi sarcoma, but it can be triggered by a weakened immune system.

Skin cancers are screened by having regular skin exams and watching for changes in moles or bumps. Even when lesions are not cancer, they could become malignant if left untreated, so being examined regularly by a medical provider is a good idea. If something looks like a potential issue, chances are good it can be biopsied or treated in the examination room. (See Question 23—How does cancer screening work?) For a more serious diagnosis like melanoma, treatments like surgery, radiation, or targeted therapy drugs might be necessary.

Breast Cancer—Breast cancer is the most common cancer diagnosis in women in the United States (aside from skin cancer). Although it is very rare, it can also affect men. Risk factors include age, menstrual and reproductive history, family history, genetics, and lifestyle factors. Most breast cancers are adenocarcinomas, tumors that develop in the milk ducts (ductal carcinoma) or milk glands (lobular carcinoma) of the breast.

Around 20 percent of breast cancer diagnoses will be ductal carcinoma in situ (DCIS) which means "in its original place." This is considered a noninvasive or pre-invasive cancer because the cancer cells have not spread out into the surrounding breast tissue. Treatment for DCIS has an excellent success rate.

However, most breast cancers are classified as invasive or infiltrating, meaning the cancer has spread into nearby tissue and has the potential to metastasize. The most common form is invasive ductal carcinoma (IDC), also referred to as breast cancer of no special type (NST). This cancer represents about 80 percent of breast cancer diagnoses in the United States. There are many rarer subtypes of IDC defined by where and how the cancer cells are growing. Invasive lobular carcinoma (ILC) is the second most common type of breast cancer, representing about 10 to 15 percent of invasive breast cancer cases. In ILC, the tumor, which originates in the milk glands, or lobules, is harder to detect and can sometimes affect both breasts.

Most women diagnosed with breast cancer do not have any family history of the disease. However, a small percentage (less than 10 percent) carry inherited genetic mutations that significantly raise their risk. The most well known of these are the BRCA1 and BRCA2 mutations, which can increase the likelihood of developing breast, ovarian, and other cancers.

Once a diagnosis of breast cancer is made, the tumor's cells are tested for the presence of certain proteins and receptors to help determine the optimal course of treatment. Some tumor cells harness hormones and growth factors to help them multiply, so if they have receptors that allow them to use estrogen (ER), or progesterone (PR), they are hormone receptor positive and can be treated with therapies that block those hormones. If tests show the tumor is producing too much of a growth-promoting protein called human epidermal growth factor receptor 2 (HER2), certain targeted therapy drugs can reverse its effects.

If these three tests come back negative, the cancer is called triple-negative breast cancer. The hormone therapies and drugs that exploit these receptor mechanisms are no longer an option. Triple-negative breast cancer accounts for about 10 to 20 percent of all breast cancer cases and tends to be aggressive and more likely to recur.

Breast cancer is screened using breast palpation to look for lumps, and imaging such as mammography, ultrasound, and MRI. (See Question 23—How does cancer screening work?) Treatment usually involves surgery, radiation, hormone therapy, or chemotherapy.

Prostate cancer—Prostate cancer is the most common cancer diagnosis in men in the United States (aside from skin cancer). Risk factors for prostate cancer include age, family history, race, and lifestyle factors. The prostate is a small gland located between the bladder and the rectum. It stores and secretes part of what makes up seminal fluid, which is essential for sperm movement and survival. Nearly all prostate cancers are adenocarcinomas and are very slow growing and slow to spread. If prostate cancer does metastasize, it usually spreads to the nearby lymph nodes. Prostate cancer is twice as likely to occur if an immediate blood relative, such as a father or brother, has had it.

There are possible pre-cancerous conditions of the prostate which, although they do not usually become cancerous themselves, can raise the risk of developing cancer in the future. Prostatic intraepithelial neoplasia (PIN) and proliferative inflammatory atrophy (PIA) involve the cells of the prostate developing an abnormal appearance or showing signs of inflammation.

Prostate cancer is commonly screened with a blood test called a prostate-specific antigen (PSA) test. Elevated levels of PSA could indicate prostate cancer. (See Question 23—How does cancer screening work?) Treatments include surgery and radiation therapy. Because it is such a slow-growing cancer, and treatment comes with many risks, treatment is not always recommended.

Lung—Lung cancer is the leading cause of cancer death in the United States, according to the ACS. This is because it is difficult to diagnose and can only be seen with medical imaging. The five-year survival rate is only 10 to 15 percent because by the time lung cancer is diagnosed, it is almost always quite advanced. People who use or have used tobacco products, or who have been exposed to radon, asbestos, or secondhand smoke, are at an increased risk of lung cancer.

Non-small cell lung cancer (NSCLC) accounts for over 80 percent of all lung cancers. Adenocarcinoma, squamous cell carcinoma, and large cell carcinoma are the three main subtypes of NSCLC. Lung adenocarcinoma occurs in the mucus-secreting cells that line the lungs. It is the most common form of lung cancer. Squamous cell carcinoma tends to develop near the center of the lungs, in the flat cells that line the main airways. Large cell carcinomas are fast-growing tumors that can appear anywhere in the lungs.

Small cell lung cancer (SCLC) is less common and more aggressive. It usually occurs in people who have smoked heavily and for a long time. It often recurs even though it responds well to chemotherapy and radiation.

Because imaging presents its own risks, low-dose computed tomography (low-dose CT or LDCT) scans are usually recommended for people at higher risk, like long-term smokers. (See Question 23—How does cancer screening work?) Lung cancer is treated with surgery, chemotherapy, radiation, immunotherapy, or targeted therapy, or often a combination of these.

Colon and Rectum—Colon, rectal, colorectal, or bowel cancer are all cancers of the large intestine. These cancers, grouped together, are the fourth most common cancer diagnosis in the United States (not counting skin cancer). Recent statistics show that colorectal cancer has become the leading cause of cancer death for men under the age of fifty. Colorectal cancer risk factors include age, family history, and lifestyle factors.

Colorectal cancers begin as polyps, growths that appear on the lining of the large intestine. Polyps are common and mostly benign, but if there are more than three, if a single polyp is very large, or if it shows signs of abnormal looking cells, there is an increased risk of it turning into cancer.

Adenocarcinoma, cancer of the mucus-secreting epithelial cells, is the most common form of colorectal cancer. The tumor can grow and penetrate the colon wall which brings it in contact with blood and lymph vessels. Some subtypes are more aggressive than others, such as signet ring and mucinous adenocarcinoma.

Colorectal cancers can be screened using tests like fecal occult blood tests, or DNA stool tests, which check the stool for signs of cancer. Different kinds of endoscopy can be used to find abnormal tissue and collect samples. (See Question 23—How does cancer screening work?) Colorectal cancer treatment usually involves surgery, radiation, chemotherapy, and targeted therapy, depending on the location and stage of the cancer.

More than half of all cancer types are considered rare, meaning they occur in fewer than six cases per 100,000 people per year. Rare cancers account for about 20 to 25 percent of all cancer diagnoses. And while these are individually uncommon, rare cancers present challenges because there is limited research, and specialists are harder to find.

No organs or tissues are completely immune to cancer, but some parts of the body are less likely to be affected than others. For example, the heart is a muscle made up of cells that stop dividing early in the body's development. As time goes on, they grow in size but not in number. For this reason, the heart is incapable of repairing itself by making more new cells in the same way bone or skin tissue would. This makes it particularly vulnerable to damage and disease. But less cell division also means less opportunity for DNA mutations or replication errors, so the heart is simply not prone to developing tumors.

Metastasis to skeletal muscle tissue is also rare, even though it is such a large percentage of the body's mass. Research suggests that the environment, already acidic and containing high levels of antioxidant enzymes, is simply not conducive to cancer cells looking for a site to metastasize.

Some other cancers such as appendix and spleen are extremely rare. It is not clear why those organs seem less likely to develop malignancies but understanding this could help in developing treatment for more common cancers.

10. How long have we known about cancer and how was it treated in the past?

Cancer is not a modern disease. Fossilized cancerous tumors have been found in the bones of dinosaurs. Some of the oldest evidence of cancer in humans was found in 1.7-million-year-old prehistoric remains. The earliest written references to the disease appear in ancient records such as the Babylonian *Code of Hammurabi* and the Chinese *Rites of the Zhou Dynasty*. The Edwin Smith Papyrus, a copy of a medical text dating back to around 3000 BC, described different kinds of tumors and instructions for their removal, with surgery or cauterization. The texts even describe late-stage breast cancer for which the medical advice is "there is nothing."

Hippocrates, a Greek physician who lived around 400 BC, first used the term "karkinos," meaning crab, to describe the disease because of the way tumors can radiate out into the tissues like a crab's legs. The disease became known in Latin as "cancer." Known as the "Father of Medicine," Hippocrates was the first to recognize the difference between malignant and benign tumors. He was ahead of his time in raising ethical standards for the practice of medicine, as well as placing the study of medicine in the realm of science rather than superstition.

However, he also theorized that cancer was caused by an imbalance of "humors" in the body, which consisted of blood, phlegm, yellow bile, and black bile. This theory was accepted for 1300 years. The Greek philosopher and physician Galen was the first to use the term "oncos" to refer to a mass or swelling, and the term "oncology" now describes the whole field of study.

During the medieval period in Europe, advances in medical knowledge slowed partly because the church banned the scientific study of the human body, including autopsies. Non-surgical treatments ranged from the unpleasant to the outright toxic, including fox lungs and arsenic. In the Middle East, physicians like Rhazes and Avenzoar continued to study and compile the ancient Greek and Roman texts, and are credited with being among the first to systematically classify diseases, as well as test surgical procedures and experimental treatments on animals. After the crusades, their writings were translated and brought back to Europe.

During the Renaissance, scientists began using the scientific method, which relied on observation, hypothesis, and experimentation. Andreas Vesalius founded the modern study of anatomy as he dissected and made careful studies of the human body. He used the corpses of executed criminals, as well as bodies obtained in much less straightforward ways. Vesalius changed the landscape of medicine when he demonstrated that the human body was made up of systems and organs and not controlled by "humors."

Throughout the centuries, scientists and physicians have theorized broadly about the causes of cancer. In the fifteenth century, Paracelsus hypothesized that cancer was caused by harmful substances in the bloodstream. In the eighteenth century, Giovanni Morgagni of Padua began performing autopsies specifically so he could isolate the causes of various diseases. His anatomical dissections and observations laid the foundation for the study of pathology and oncology. At this time, many scientists were correlating environmental exposure to cancer, notably English surgeon Percival Pott, who observed the relationship between soot and cancer of the scrotum among London's chimney sweeps.

Scientists also pursued the idea that cancer could run in families. In the nineteenth century, Austrian monk and biologist Gregor Mendel did his pioneering work experimenting with inherited traits and is regarded as the founder of scientific genetics. Hilario de Gouvea, a Brazilian ophthalmologist, was the first to document that cancer risk could be inherited, as in the case of retinoblastoma, a malignant eye tumor.

During this time, the development of the modern microscope ushered in huge advances in cellular biology and allowed tumors to be studied in greater detail. Swiss chemist Friedrich Miescher identified something in the nucleus of cells which was not a protein as he had expected. He called it "nuclein." German biochemist Albrecht Kossel soon identified it as a nucleic acid and gave it its chemical name, deoxyribonucleic acid, or DNA. Kossel also identified its nucleotide bases, for which he was awarded a Nobel Prize. It would still be some time before the molecular structure of cancer and genetics were scientifically connected.

German biologist Rudolf Virchow realized that not only was cancer made up of "corrupted cells," it originated from normal cells. He was the first to note a connection between cancer and inflammation. His work helped the field of scientific oncology take off.

At the beginning of the twentieth century, German biologist Theodor Boveri proposed the chromosome theory of inheritance, that uncontrolled cellular proliferation was related to changes in the chromosomes, and that cancer originated from a single cell.

The early twentieth century also saw great advances in identifying viruses that can cause cancer. American pathologist Peyton Rous was the first to isolate a cancer-causing retrovirus which he called the Rous Sarcoma Virus. Its ability to quickly induce cancer in a normal cell allowed researchers to study cancer on a molecular level for the first time. It led many at the time to believe cancer was caused by viruses, but we know now that only about 12 percent of cancers are associated with viral infection.

During this time, the observational and mathematical science of epidemiology was evolving, and in 1950, Sir Austin Hill and Sir Richard Doll demonstrated a causal link between tobacco smoking and cancer.

In 1953, the collective work of James Watson, Francis Crick, Maurice Wilkins, and Rosalind Franklin led to the discovery of DNA's double helix structure. This breakthrough revealed how genes encode and replicate information and clarified our knowledge of hereditary diseases. It paved the way for understanding the mechanisms of mutations and DNA repair, as well as how cancer develops on a molecular level. Scientists recognized that trauma or illness, environmental exposure, viruses, inflammation, and family history, all the theories about what caused cancer, had a common denominator: damage to the DNA.

It is easy to dismiss early cancer treatments as quackery or butchery, but some of them ultimately became the basis for modern therapies. Opium and its derivatives are still used today for pain relief, many herbs and plants are the basis of chemicals we use in modern drugs, and the first records of treating breast cancer by mastectomy, or surgically removing the breast, date back to the first centuries AD.

Although surgery had been practiced for thousands of years, surgeons were still hindered by the issues of bleeding, pain, and infection which made it a treatment of last resort. But the introduction of general anesthesia in the nineteenth century revolutionized surgery, which is still considered a first-line cancer treatment today. The development of anesthesia bought the surgeon more time and allowed for more complicated, finely tuned procedures.

Around this time, Louis Pasteur and Joseph Lister discovered that bacteria were the origin of infection, and the advent of antiseptic surgery and sterilization further improved chances of survival. American surgeon William Halsted performed the first radical mastectomy during this time, a disfiguring procedure which remained the standard until late into the 1970s. His approach was to remove as much tissue as possible to control the disease, but it was not yet recognized that the determining factor in surviving breast cancer was metastasis, not tumor growth. He is credited, though, with developing the practice of rigorous surgical prep, including scrubbing, and wearing gowns and gloves, one of the reasons why modern surgery is safe, effective, and reliable.

The concept of immunotherapy goes back to the nineteenth century, when William Coley, an American surgeon, observed the relationship between post-surgical infection and cancer regression in his patients. It was as if their immune system, once activated by the infection, was attacking the cancer as well. He concluded that generating an immune response could successfully shrink a tumor and administered solutions of bacteria to stimulate this response. It was often effective, but sometimes fatal. Ultimately, it led scientists to advance the idea that the immune system was capable of fighting cancer. They had no idea why it was working, and it did not work for every patient, so the field of immunotherapy went out of favor. Coley's daughter, Helen Coley Nauts, would go on to consolidate his research and help found the Cancer Research Institute in 1953, to promote the study of cancer immunity.

At the end of the nineteenth century, the discoveries of x-rays by Wilhelm Röntgen, and radium by Marie and Pierre Curie, quickly ushered in the use of radiation therapy and transformed the way cancer was treated.

Paul Erlich, a German physician, experimented with dyes that only reacted with certain cells, positing that drugs could be developed that would only target cancer cells. After the First World War, doctors noticed that the bone marrow of soldiers being treated for exposure to mustard gas was affected very differently from other cells in the body. By the 1940s, scientists realized mustard gas was targeting fast-growing cells and could be used to fight cancer, effectively becoming the basis for modern chemotherapy.

Pathologist Sidney Farber began successfully treating children with leukemia with antimetabolites, drugs that block metabolic pathways. This research opened the door for many new treatments such as taxanes and platinum complexes. It was soon determined that chemotherapy drugs, some of which are still in use today, worked better in combinations than individually.

The first successful bone marrow, or stem cell, transplant was performed in the 1950s by E. Donnall Thomas. Since then, the creation of a donor registry has made matching more efficient and saved many lives.

Once the structure of DNA was discovered, research began in earnest into how genetic mutations drove cancer development. American biochemist Bruce Ames developed the Ames Test in 1973, which is used to test chemicals for their mutagenic or carcinogenic potential. In 1977, Frederick Sanger developed a technique to determine the exact sequence of bases in a DNA molecule, a fast, accurate, and reliable method still used today. This kind of sequencing led to the discovery of more proto-oncogenes, oncogenes, and tumor suppressor genes. Twenty years later, the breast cancer gene BRCA1 was identified, cloned, and sequenced, marking a huge leap in being able to personalize and target treatment. Sequencing genes associated with cancer has helped in identifying risk factors and improving cancer prevention.

The Human Genome Project is perhaps the most ambitious research endeavor of the twentieth century. This monumental scientific undertaking officially started in 1990 and was completed in 2003, having achieved the first sequence of the entire human genome, over 3 billion nucleotides. It also promoted sharing scientific data, brought biomedical ethics to the forefront, and drove the improvement of genomic sequencing technologies. It launched the field of cancer genomics, which has resulted in unprecedented progress and pace in the twenty-first century. Two years later, The Cancer Genome Atlas project was launched with the purpose of cataloging all genomic changes in all human cancers, a comprehensive, systematic, large-scale, data-sharing effort.

The Human Genome Project also ushered in the era of genetic engineering in cancer treatment, specifically for immunotherapy. Monoclonal antibodies were first created in the 1970s by César Milstein and Georges Köhler. The first monoclonal antibody therapy for cancer was approved in 1986. Since then, many therapies have been engineered to target specific cancers, manipulate or stimulate an immune system response, and transport and bind cancer drugs directly to the tumor.

Although vaccines have existed since the nineteenth century, some cancer vaccines have now been developed specifically to prevent viral infections that increase cancer risk, such as Hepatitis B (HBV) and human papillomavirus (HPV). And with current genetic technology, many therapeutic cancer vaccines are being developed that can target the overexpressed proteins on an individual tumor.

In 2013, cancer immunotherapy was *Science* magazine's "Breakthrough of the Year." In 2018, James Allison and Tasuku Honjo received the Nobel Prize for their work on immunotherapy and discovering how and why the immune system can be harnessed to fight cancer. In 2017, the Food and Drug Administration (FDA) approved the first gene therapy for cancer, a procedure which involves transferring new genetic material into the cells to correct an abnormal gene. In the last decade, many breakthroughs in cancer research have come in the form of more targeted treatments, and the future direction of cancer research will focus even more on precision, or personalized, medicine. (See Question 46—What is the future of cancer research?)

11. What is the economic burden of cancer?

Cancer is the second leading cause of death worldwide. By 2040, new annual cancer cases are expected to rise to 30.2 million, with deaths reaching 16.3 million. This growing burden affects individuals, families, health care systems, and economies. The economic impact includes both direct and indirect costs, straining not only patients but society as a whole. Despite medical advances, progress in cancer treatment has not kept pace with the rising incidence of the disease, making its economic toll increasingly difficult to manage.

Although cancer death rates are declining, the total number of deaths continues to rise due to global population growth and aging. Age is the biggest risk factor for cancer. According to the US Census Bureau, the number of Americans over sixty-five will double by 2060, and by 2035, older adults will outnumber children for the first time in United States history.

The direct medical costs of cancer include procedures and treatment services, cancer drugs and supporting medications, hospitalization, diagnostic tests, alternative therapies, follow-up visits, rehabilitation, palliative, and supportive care. Cancer costs vary depending on the type of cancer and how early it is diagnosed, but they peak during end-of-life care. Indirect costs of cancer include lost income, reduced productivity, caregiver and home care expenses, and long-term disability.

In the United States, these costs are shared among private insurers, public health care programs like Medicare and Medicaid, and the patients themselves. According to the American Cancer Society (ACS), in 2018, cancer patients paid $5.6 billion out of pocket for their cancer treatments. Cancer is one of the most expensive conditions to treat, with many people requiring treatment for months or years.

In 2013, the term "financial toxicity" was coined by oncologists at Duke Cancer Center to describe the financial and emotional impact of the medical expenses associated with cancer. Financial toxicity relates to both objective financial burdens, and subjective financial distress. A 2021 ACS survey revealed a quarter of their respondents delayed or cancelled care because of cost, even though 98 percent of responders had health care coverage at the time they accumulated their medical debt.

And as treatments improve and more people survive their cancer, they face the financial consequences of survivorship, as they will require a lifetime of monitoring and imaging, treatment for the long-term toxicity of their cancer therapy, and lost productivity. Survivors of pediatric cancer are at especially high risk of developing other chronic physical and mental health issues over their lifetime. Caregivers also bear physical, emotional, and financial burdens, and often go unsupported. One of the most significant intangible costs of cancer is the loss of quality of life.

Cancer's financial impact does not affect everyone equally. The 2020 edition of the American Cancer Society's Cancer Action Network (ACS CAN), *The Costs of Cancer*, revealed that patients who are young, less educated, people of color, or from low-income backgrounds are more likely to face financial hardship.

The National Cancer Institute (NCI) estimated cancer-related healthcare spending at $208.9 billion in 2020, projected to increase to $245 billion by 2030. This growing demand will strain health care systems, raise insurance premiums, and burden public budgets. On a macroeconomic level, cancer affects economic growth through loss of workforce and economic productivity, unemployment, and capital investment reductions. A 2023 analytical modeling study published in the *Journal of the American Medical Association Oncology* estimated that between 2020 and 2050, cancer will cost the world's economy $25.2 trillion in international dollars.

While high-income countries bear the largest economic costs, low- and middle-income countries, which see 75 percent of world cancer deaths, suffer the greatest health burden due to limited access to care. A World Health Organization (WHO) survey of 115 countries revealed that a majority of these have not adequately prioritized the future costs of cancer care.

Efforts to address cancer's economic impact face political and logistical challenges. A 2023 study published in *The Lancet Oncology* reported that between 2016 and 2020, the United States provided 57.3 percent of the total funding for cancer research, globally. Federal taxes pay for research, government regulation, and medical care, through federally funded public health programs like Medicare and Medicaid. However, political agendas influence how research and health care policies are shaped and funded.

Developing new cancer drugs is costly and slow. It can take twelve to fifteen years and over $2.3 billion to bring a new drug to market, from the discovery phase to Food and Drug Administration (FDA) approval. To develop a new drug, scientists identify a potential drug compound which is first tested in model systems to help predict how the therapy will perform in humans. Preclinical assessments using cellular (in vitro) and animal (in vivo) studies help determine the drug's potential for toxicity and adverse reactions. Before human testing can begin, the manufacturer submits an Investigational New Drug (IND) application to the FDA for review. Following this, the drug undergoes phased clinical trials, which can take between two and eight years to complete.

Clinical trials are generally broken down into four phases. Phase I trials test for safety and dosage on a very small group of patients. Phase II trials further evaluate the safety of the drug and focus on effectiveness. Phase III trials compare the new treatment against existing standard of care in a larger population. At this point, when the drug has demonstrated clear benefits and acceptable risks, a New Drug Application (NDA) is submitted to the FDA for approval. Once a drug is approved, it is marketed and sold. Phase IV trials provide post-marketing surveillance, monitoring safety, and collecting further information about long-term benefits and side effects. Rare or delayed side effects can lead to warnings or withdrawal. But if the drug shows it is effective against other cancers, it may receive expanded approval for new uses.

Aside from the sheer cost and complexity involved in running these trials, there are significant challenges. The overall failure rate for oncology drug development is quite high. A 2023 report in the *International Journal of Cancer* estimated that only about 5 percent of drug candidates entering clinical trials eventually gained FDA approval. Enrollment in cancer clinical trials is one of the biggest challenges. Participation rates are very low, ranging from 3 to 16 percent, which cause trials to be extended, delaying research, and further increasing costs.

Because of these high costs, the process depends on partnership with industry, and close to 75 percent of United States funding for clinical trials comes from private companies including pharmaceutical, biotech, and startups. With that kind of investment, the corporate sector is less inclined to share clinical trial results, even though the data would help other researchers and physicians, and it would speed up the progress against cancer. The FDA Amendment Act of 2007 mandates that certain clinical trials must report on their findings. But according to a 2017 study published in the journal *Trials*, many still fail to comply within the required timeframe.

Progress can also be undermined when industries' interests are at odds with what is best for public health. Politicians are heavily influenced by interest groups and lobbyists, and political and industry influence can potentially prioritize commercial interests over medical access or environmental safety. So, sometimes the profit motive can displace public welfare.

Cancer itself has become an industry that generates billions of dollars every year. The United States oncology market size was valued at $147 billion in 2022, and is anticipated to reach $312 billion by 2032, according to some market research firms. Most accelerated drug approvals from the FDA go to cancer treatments, which means the drugs reach patients faster. But a study published in the *Journal of the American Medical Association* revealed that fewer than half of these drugs showed a clinical benefit after five years. Critics argue that treating cancer can be profitable, even when it is not very effective, and that making cancer treatments is more profitable than making a cure.

So, is it possible to stop treating cancer like big business or a political football without stifling the speed and scope of innovation? Health policies must be guided by scientific evidence and made within the best interests of public welfare. Transparency, accountability, and nonprofit research funding are vital. Data sharing and collaboration can reduce costs and duplication of effort, speeding up progress.

Prevention offers the highest return on investment. A 2019 global study published in *The Lancet* found that 44.4 percent of cancer deaths worldwide were attributable to modifiable risk factors like smoking, infection, and obesity. The problem with prevention is that governments tend to be more reactive than proactive, but targeting key risk factors could result in massive economic and societal dividends. Public health efforts should promote healthy lifestyles, screening programs, and early detection, which are far less expensive than treating late-stage disease. Telehealth and digital tools can expand access to preventive care and counseling. Governments also have the regulatory power to create and enforce safety standards when it comes to occupational and environmental exposure.

Understanding the scope of cancer's burden is the first step. Cancer registries like the NCI's Surveillance, Epidemiology, and End Results (SEER) program, and the Centers for Disease Control and Prevention's (CDC's) National Program of Cancer Registries (NPCR), track and collect data on cancer incidence which can help guide governments in creating policies, determining where and how resources should be allocated, maximizing investments in research and development, promoting innovation, and building health care systems that will meet anticipated needs.

Efficient resource allocation is essential because research, clinical trials, awareness campaigns, and health initiatives are expensive. The NCI, which was created in 1937 to promote cancer research, is the largest funder of cancer research in the world. The NCI's 2024 budget was $7.22 billion, to be used for research, training, and information dissemination. Initiatives like the US Cancer Moonshot aim to reduce cancer death rates by 50 percent over twenty-five years. International efforts, such as the European Code Against Cancer and WHO's Global Action Plan, also support prevention and access to care.

At the individual level, there are countless programs available in the United States that play a role in preventing cancer and improving health outcomes for patients. There are many support services that offer free or low-cost cancer screening, vaccinations, and health and nutrition counseling. Many employers are required by law to accommodate people undergoing cancer treatment. The Department of Labor lists various federal and state protections and employer-provided leave benefits that might be available to cancer patients and their care givers. The NCI offers a database called "Organizations that Offer Support." Many organizations, like the Patient Advocate Foundation and Cancer Care, offer financial assistance services, and many pharmaceutical companies offer free or discounted medication to eligible patients. These and many other nonprofits and foundations exist to help patients navigate their cancer experience. (See Question 20—What organizations and public health initiatives exist, and how can they help prevent cancer?)

Cancer Causes, Risk Factors, and Prevention

12. What causes cancer?

Cancer is caused by disruptions in normal cell growth, mutations, which can be triggered by a wide range of substances or biological processes. A few cancers can easily be attributed to specific risk factors, but for many, the exact causes are complex and still poorly understood. Some cancers are caused by inherited genes, but most cancers are sporadic, which means they occur at some point due to random genetic mutations, or mutations precipitated by exposure to carcinogens, medical conditions, or infections. (See Question 18—What are carcinogens?)

The terms "cause" and "risk factor" are often used together but are not always interchangeable. A cause is responsible for initiating the disease or promoting its growth, whereas a risk factor is a characteristic, condition, or behavior that increases the probability of developing it. For example, age is one of the biggest risk factors when it comes to cancer. The longer people live, the more likely they are to develop the disease. But age does not cause cancer.

So, all causal factors are also risk factors, but not all risk factors are causal. On top of that, cause and risk are difficult to confirm and are often simply inferred. A variety of factors can work simultaneously or in sequence to initiate and promote the disease. Their effects can be cumulative as well as synergistic, and they vary in terms of degree. For example, an obese smoker will be at a higher risk than someone who is just obese. Risk often depends on the length and extent of the exposure. In addition, cancer can appear between five and forty years after the initial mutation, which makes pinpointing its causes extremely tricky. (See Question 4—What role does mutation play in cancer development?)

Only 5 to 10 percent of cancers are hereditary or related to family history. In these cases, the disease is caused by an inherited mutation that is "preloaded" in the cells. The rest of cancer cases arise from mutations that are acquired over the life of an individual. Some cancer-causing mutations are due to outside factors such as exposure to chemical, physical, or biological agents. Other mutations can happen inside the body, triggered by chronic inflammation, hormones, and a variety of medical conditions.

Chemical agents are things we are exposed to every day, environmentally, occupationally, and through lifestyle choices. Most chemical agents are present in nature and pose no significant risk. The danger depends on the extent of the exposure. Arsenic, for example, is a highly toxic natural element present in many chemical compounds. Excessive exposure and contamination happen due to runoff from mining, agriculture, and coal burning power plants, and, until recently, was present in pressure treated lumber and certain pesticides. It has been found in a variety of things we consume, including seafood, rice, and drinking water. Arsenic can cause direct damage to DNA and has been linked to lung, bladder, and skin cancer, among others.

Tobacco smoke is a complex combination of chemicals, which includes arsenic, formaldehyde, lead, benzene, carbon monoxide, polonium-210, and vinyl chloride. These carcinogens come from the tobacco itself, additives that are combined with it, and chemicals produced by burning. Tobacco smoke is particularly dangerous because it goes directly and deeply into the lungs. Since there are so many different chemicals in it, tobacco can induce cancer in many ways. Tobacco smoke causes physical damage to the lungs, generates mutations in DNA, causes oxidative stress in the cells, and creates a huge burden on the immune system, resulting in chronic inflammation. Smoking causes at least sixteen different types of cancer, including lung, colorectal, mouth and throat, and pancreatic.

Asbestos is a fibrous material that is resistant to heat and corrosion. Exposure happens through environmental or occupational contact like construction, mining, and manufacturing. It is less common now that it is heavily regulated, but can still be found in some products made before 1900, or houses built before 1980. When asbestos is disturbed, its tiny fibers are released into the air. When inhaled, they become trapped and cause scarring, chronic inflammation, and direct damage to DNA.

Asbestos exposure is associated with mesothelioma, a cancer that affects the lining of the internal organs, and is also linked to lung, larynx, and ovarian cancer. Between 80 and 90 percent of mesotheliomas are caused by asbestos but this rare cancer is slow to develop which is why people are still being diagnosed with it twenty to forty years after exposure. Johnson & Johnson, a health care company, is currently the subject of lawsuits that claim the company's talcum powder led to ovarian cancer and mesothelioma. While talc itself cannot cause cancer, talc and asbestos frequently occur near each other in nature and contamination can happen during mining.

Formaldehyde is another chemical used in industry and building. It is found in household products, as a preservative in cosmetics and food, and in air pollution and smoke. Heavy exposure is more likely to happen to people in occupational settings like laboratory technicians or embalmers. It can be absorbed mostly by inhaling, but also ingesting, or through the skin. Formaldehyde has been linked to leukemia, and nose and throat cancers.

Polychlorinated biphenyls (PCBs) are synthetic chemicals that were used in industrial and commercial products to make them more durable and flame retardant. Banned in 1976, they can still be found in old plastics, capacitors, and transformers. Aside from being associated with liver, pancreatic, and testicular cancer, PCBs are also linked to skin conditions and birth defects.

Air pollutants like diesel exhaust, gasoline fumes, and factory emissions all contain cancer-causing chemicals such as soot particles and combustion byproducts, polycyclic aromatic hydrocarbons (PAHs), and benzene. Exposure to air pollution varies but is highest in cities and industrial areas. Length and extent of exposure have the most effect on risk. Cancers linked with these chemicals include leukemia, lung, skin, and bladder cancer.

Perfluoroalkyl and polyfluoroalkyl substances (PFAs), and perfluorooctanoic acids (PFOAs) are a category of synthetic molecules that are added to products like plastics, non-stick cookware, paint, and carpeting. They have been called "forever chemicals" because they can leach from packaging and contaminate products like food, cosmetics, and household cleaners, and take a very long time to break down. These chemicals are endocrine disruptors, meaning they interfere with the way hormones work in the body. They have been linked to kidney and testicular cancer.

Bisphenol-A, or BPA, is an endocrine disruptor that mimics estrogen. It is found in many plastic products and some aluminum cans. Some research has shown it can seep into foods. Although the Food and Drug Administration (FDA) states that BPA is safe at current low levels, studies suggest potential risks in relation to hormone-sensitive cancers. More data is needed to know for sure.

Microplastics are plastic particles less than 5 millimeters in diameter. They come from industrial production as well as the breakdown of larger plastic items. Their widespread presence raises concerns about how they interact with both the environment and the human body. Although the World Health Organization (WHO) states there is not yet enough evidence to directly link microplastics to cancer in humans, these tiny particles have been shown to promote oxidative stress and chronic inflammation, which are well-known factors in cancer development. Studies are increasingly discovering microplastics in human tissue and organs, including the brain.

All alcohol contains ethanol, which is broken down in the body into acetaldehyde. Most of this conversion process occurs in the liver, and when acetaldehyde builds up in the system it can cause direct damage to DNA. This damage to the liver can result in cirrhosis, which increases the risk of liver cancer. Alcohol is also associated with mouth and throat, esophageal, stomach, and colorectal cancers because it can be an irritant to the tissues of the digestive system. It causes oxidative stress and can also act as a solvent to help other harmful chemicals penetrate the cell lining. These risks increase with increased consumption. Alcohol also raises circulating estrogen levels in the body which is why it can increase the risk of breast cancer.

The WHO states there is convincing evidence that processed (smoked, salted, or cured) meats can cause cancer because of the chemical compounds they contain. Nitrites and nitrates are used by manufacturers to preserve meats like deli meats, hot dogs, sausages, jerky, and bacon. These chemicals, and others found in salt preserved foods like salted fish, lead to the formation of cancer-causing compounds called N-nitroso-compounds (NOC).

Meat in general, and red meat especially, contains heme iron which, in large amounts, could trigger oxidative reactions and promote tumorigenesis. Cooking foods at high temperatures such as deep frying and grilling produces chemicals from the searing called acrylamides and heterocyclic aromatic amines. These chemicals have been associated with the development of stomach, pancreatic, and colorectal cancer. Ultra-processed foods have been increasingly associated with cancer risk because they generally contain one or more of these cancer-causing chemicals as well as dyes, additives, sugars, and sodium which cause inflammation and promote obesity.

Physical agents like radiation can cause cancer because they directly damage DNA. Ionizing radiation like x-rays or gamma rays, is a high-frequency radiation that has enough energy to ionize (or knock an electron out of) an atom or molecule, thereby causing breaks in DNA. It can occur in nature in the form of radioactive elements in the ground, and cosmic rays from outer space. The largest source of background radiation comes from radon gas. In tightly insulated buildings it can accumulate and reach dangerous levels of concentration. High levels of radon are also found in uranium mines. Radon is a gas that decays quickly and releases small radioactive particles which, when inhaled, damage the cells lining the lungs. It is the number one cause of lung cancer in nonsmokers.

Most studies on radiation and cancer focus on unusually high levels of exposure, such as survivors of atomic bombs in Japan, Chernobyl, and people who were exposed to above ground nuclear testing. The effects of these levels are obvious, and result in many types of cancer, including leukemia and thyroid cancer. It is harder to study the effects of the radiation used in medical imaging like x-rays and CT scans. These types of radiation levels are equivalent to background radiation. According to the FDA, which regulates radiation levels in medical imaging, the cancer risk is very low.

Radiation therapy used to treat cancer has been linked with an increased risk of leukemia, thyroid, and breast cancer, a risk that is weighed against potential benefits. This risk is also low overall, and depends on the dose, the part of the body, the patient's age, and whether other potentially mutagenic treatments are being used.

Ultraviolet (UV) radiation has less energy than ionizing radiation. Most UV rays cannot penetrate deeply into the body, but they can affect the skin. UV exposure can cause skin cancer like basal and squamous cell carcinoma, melanoma, and melanoma of the eye. The sun is the main source of UV radiation exposure, and a sunburn is essentially a radiation burn. It is an unmistakable sign that the skin cells have been damaged all the way down to their DNA.

UVA rays are the weakest and make up about 95 percent of the sun's radiation. Long-term exposure can cause skin damage and aging and is thought to play a role in some skin cancers. UVB rays can damage DNA in the cells directly and are the main cause of sunburn and skin cancer. UV rays can also come from artificial sources such as tanning beds, black-light lamps, plasma torches, and welding arcs. Studies show people who use tanning beds have an increased risk of skin cancer.

Biological agents can cause cancer by triggering chronic inflammation and disrupting normal cell regulation. Aspergillus is a kind of mold that produces a mycotoxin called aflatoxin. It grows on crops like corn, peanuts, and tree nuts. Exposure to this toxin comes from eating contaminated plants, or meat from animals that have fed on contaminated plants. The United States and many other countries test and treat foods for aflatoxins, but outbreaks still happen in developing countries. Aflatoxins are associated with an increased risk of liver cancer. Other naturally occurring carcinogenic plant toxins include pyrrolizidine alkaloids, which can be found in some teas, herbs, and spices.

According to the American Cancer Society (ACS), 15 to 20 percent of cancers worldwide are linked to infections caused by viruses, parasites, and bacteria. These infections can result in cancer in a variety of ways. Many cause long-term or chronic inflammation, and some suppress the immune system altogether. Some viruses insert their genes directly into a cell to reproduce, causing it to multiply uncontrollably.

Human papillomavirus (HPV) is the most common infection-related cause of cancer in the United States. HPV infections may cause genital warts but generally have mild to no symptoms. People who have long-lasting asymptomatic infections are at higher risk of developing cancer. Recent studies have found a higher incidence of head and neck cancer in young people when HPV is present. HPV can be transmitted through any intimate skin-to-skin contact. According to the National Cancer Institute (NCI), HPV is also implicated in anal, throat, penile, vaginal, and vulvar cancer.

The Epstein-Barr virus (EBV) is a type of herpes virus. It causes mononucleosis, or "mono," which is highly infectious and can be transmitted through airborne pathways or direct contact. Most people in the United States have been infected by EBV, although not everyone develops symptoms. Very few people infected with EBV will ever develop cancer, but it has been associated with an increased risk of nasopharyngeal cancer and certain kinds of lymphomas.

Hepatitis B (HBV) and Hepatitis C (HCV) are viruses that cause long-term chronic liver infections which increase the chance of developing liver cancer. These infections are spread through contact with body fluids like blood, saliva, vaginal fluid, and semen. HBV is especially associated with people with substance abuse issues who share needles.

The Kaposi sarcoma-associated herpesvirus (KSHV), also known as the human herpesvirus 8 (HHV-8), causes an infection which can lead to a rare soft tissue cancer called Kaposi's sarcoma. It is often linked to the human immunodeficiency virus (HIV), both of which can be transmitted through body fluids during sexual contact, blood transfusion and transplants, and from a mother to her infant during birth. HIV itself increases the risk of getting several types of cancer because it weakens the immune system and makes infections like HHV-8 harder to fight. HIV is also associated with cervical cancer and non-Hodgkin lymphoma.

Certain bacterial infections can lead to cancer. Helicobacter pylori (H pylori) is a bacterial infection of the stomach that can be transmitted through contaminated food and water, or with mouth-to-mouth contact. The infection causes ulcers and inflammation and increases the risk of stomach cancer. Chlamydia trachomatis is a sexually transmitted infection that affects the reproductive organs. Studies suggest that chlamydia might increase the risk of cervical cancer, especially in women who are also positive for HPV. Chlamydia can lead to pelvic inflammatory disease which is a risk factor for ovarian cancer.

Parasites that live inside the human body can also raise the risk of developing cancer. Although rarely found in the United States, they are still common elsewhere in the world. Liver flukes are flat worms that come from eating raw or undercooked freshwater fish. These parasites are linked to cancer of the bile ducts. Schistosoma hematoxylin is a parasite found in water. This parasitic infection called schistosomiasis has been linked to bladder cancer.

Infections that can lead to cancer can be highly contagious, but cancer itself is not contagious. One person cannot give cancer to another. There is no risk through casual or intimate contact. There is no evidence that you can get cancer from a blood transfusion.

Sometimes, cancer development is not caused by an outside source, it can be triggered inside the body, by chronic inflammation, hormones, and a variety of medical conditions.

Inflammation is a hallmark of cancer. Acute inflammation is the immune system's initial response to injury, like the redness, warmth, and swelling from a sprained ankle. It fights infection and speeds up healing. Chronic inflammation is a prolonged response to a stimulus that will not go away. The body perceives a constant attack, so it mounts a constant response. When this occurs, the immune system ends up attacking healthy tissue and causing damage inside the body. Chronic inflammation promotes cancer development by releasing too many reactive oxygen species (ROS) into the cells. These highly reactive unstable molecules are a byproduct of cellular metabolism, and their function is to act as messengers in a variety of normal biological processes. Cells contain antioxidants to counteract the negative effects of ROS. However, a buildup or imbalance of ROS can result in oxidative stress which causes DNA damage. Chronic inflammation can be caused by conditions like autoimmune disorders, cardiovascular disease, and diabetes, as well as mental health disorders, sleeplessness, and chronic stress.

Hormones and hormonal fluctuations have been linked to certain cancers such as breast, endometrial, ovarian, prostate, and thyroid. The endocrine system produces hormones which are chemical messengers that reach organs all over the body. They regulate metabolism, growth, and reproductive development. The relationship between hormones and cancer is ever evolving and complex. What is clear is that certain hormones cause cells to multiply rapidly. Rapidly multiplying cells are more likely to mutate. Hormones can also cause a tumor to grow more aggressively. Some cancers are hormone-sensitive or hormone-dependent, which means they are specifically using hormones to fuel their growth.

Some medical conditions can increase the risk of certain cancers by causing DNA damage, by creating favorable environments for cancers to grow, or simply by preventing the immune system from stopping cancer development before it starts.

Obesity heightens the risk of many chronic illnesses and is associated with thirteen types of cancer including endometrial, colorectal, liver, gallbladder, pancreas, and kidney. Body fat is part of the endocrine system and has an impact on metabolism. It is involved in the regulation of a variety of biological functions and communicates with other organs and systems through hormone signals. So, excess body fat can cause several biological mechanisms to malfunction. Obesity causes levels of growth hormones to rise, which encourages cells to multiply more rapidly. It promotes chronic inflammation, insulin resistance, and diabetes, all of which promote or fuel cancer development.

People with diabetes, especially Type II diabetes, are at an increased risk for liver, pancreatic, colorectal, endometrial, breast, and bladder cancer. Gastrointestinal conditions like Crohn's disease and ulcerative colitis increase the risk of colon cancer, and cirrhosis of the liver increases the risk of liver cancer. Damage to an organ due to chronic infection or inflammation increases the risk of cancer in that organ. A rare inflammatory disease called dermatomyositis is associated with an elevated risk of developing cancer in general.

Studies have shown that people with a history of gum disease have a greater chance of developing stomach cancer as well as the type of polyp that can lead to colon cancer.

Cryptorchidism, a condition in which one or both testicles are undescended, is one of the main risk factors for testicular cancer.

Being an organ transplant recipient also increases the risk of cancer. Drugs that suppress the immune system to prevent organ rejection weaken the immune system, which increases cancer risk. Certain post-transplant infections, such as hepatitis, can themselves lead to cancer even if the infection is successfully treated. There have been extremely rare cases of people getting cancer after receiving an organ transplant from a donor who had an undiagnosed malignancy, but there are stringent screening processes in place that minimize the risk.

13. What role do lifestyle choices play in cancer risk?

People say everything causes cancer. While it is true that many things are technically carcinogenic, the most common cancers are associated with the most common risk factors, because cancer risk is a question of degree and exposure. Statistically, it is what we are exposed to frequently, and long-term, which puts us at risk. Most people in the United States will never experience exotic parasites or atomic bombs. What they will be exposed to, every day, are their own lifestyle choices.

A global study published in *The Lancet* in 2019 found that 44.4 percent of cancer deaths worldwide were attributable to modifiable risk factors. The bad news is that people are putting themselves at risk through their own lifestyle choices. But the good news is that nearly half of cancer deaths are potentially avoidable by changing certain habits or behaviors.

Tobacco use is the leading cause of preventable death in the United States. It is the single most significant lifestyle choice that puts people at risk of cancer. Yet, according to the CDC, 28.3 million people in the United States are smokers. People say smoking helps them focus, forces them to take breaks, that it suppresses their appetite, and that it soothes and calms. Add to that the fact that nicotine is as addictive as cocaine, and it is easy to understand why people still smoke despite knowing it is bad for them.

But with 250 known harmful chemicals, at least seventy of which are known carcinogens, it is simply not worth the health risk. Beyond the cellular damage caused by the chemicals, physical damage to the lungs also precipitates chronic inflammation. Tobacco use is linked to at least sixteen different kinds of cancer, such as lung, colorectal, mouth and throat, and pancreatic. Secondhand smoke is a risk factor for non-smokers, increasing their risk of lung cancer by 20 to 30 percent.

There is less evidence that marijuana and other drugs are as carcinogenic as tobacco, but a 2024 study published in the journal *Addiction Biology*, identified cannabis as genotoxic, or capable of causing direct damage to DNA. Cannabis is also associated with an increased risk of testicular cancer in young men. Cocaine use is associated with head and neck cancer risk. Smoking, snorting, or huffing of any substance results in tissue damage and chronic inflammation over time. The biggest danger presented by illicit drugs is that they are often mixed, or cut, with toxic and carcinogenic chemicals, like phenacetin, which has been linked to renal, pelvic, and bladder cancer. Injection drug use is risky because sharing needles can lead to infections like hepatitis which increases the risk of liver cancer.

There is currently no compelling evidence that vaping is associated with cancer, but E-cigarettes still contain known carcinogens like benzene, heavy metals, and formaldehyde, albeit at much lower levels than cigarettes. Vaping is clearly less harmful than smoking, but the concern with E-cigarettes is that there is little regulation about the ingredients they might contain, and even less information about what happens when these ingredients are heated, their interactions with other chemicals, and their long-term effects.

Ultraviolet (UV) radiation exposure increases the risk of skin cancer. Spending time outdoors in sunlight and fresh air has been shown to improve physical health and mental well-being. But getting a serious sunburn is a high-risk lifestyle choice. According to the Environmental Protection Agency (EPA), the average American spends 90 percent of their time indoors. This means that getting intense or prolonged exposure to UV rays is even more likely to cause severe damage to the skin. Getting a sunburn just once every two years triples the risk of getting melanoma. Using tanning beds or booths is even more dangerous because they emit three times more UV rays than the sun, and the cancer risk increases in people under thirty-five. Being active outside is an excellent lifestyle choice, just remember to protect your skin during peak sunny hours.

From 1990 to 2019, the global incidence of cancer in younger adults increased by 79 percent, according to a study published in the *British Medical Journal Oncology*. Although the reasons for the shift are unclear, they seem to be related to what is called the "Western lifestyle," which is characterized by a modern western diet (high in ultra-processed foods, high in fats and sugar, and low in whole grains and fiber) and sedentary habits. Poor diet, obesity, physical inactivity, alcohol, and sleep deprivation are all implicated in chronic metabolic inflammation and are all cancer risk factors. These factors tend to occur in clusters, with the presence of one increasing the likelihood of the others.

Poor diet seems to be on the list of risk factors for many medical issues. A 2019 study published in *Journal of the National Cancer Institute: Cancer Spectrum* showed that an unhealthy diet was tied to 5 percent of all cancer cases in the United States. The biggest risk factors they identified were low vegetable and fruit intake, low whole grain consumption, low dietary calcium intake, high red and processed meat intake, and high intake of sugar sweetened beverages. Poor diet may influence many types of cancer, but it is most associated with colorectal and other digestive tract cancers.

Diet also relates to the gut microbiome because nutrition affects the composition and function of gut bacteria. Gastrointestinal cancers are associated with dysbiosis, the imbalance between the digestive system and the bacteria that live there. A healthy diet helps to support the immune system, and a well-functioning immune system is less likely to cause chronic inflammation. Eating charred foods or even sitting close to burning wood or charcoal increases exposure to polycyclic aromatic hydrocarbons (PAHs). Diets high in saturated fat are also associated with post-menopausal breast cancer and prostate cancer because they disrupt hormones and the endocrine system. People who make poor diet choices are also more likely to have other unhealthy habits and other underlying risk factors like obesity.

Excess body weight and obesity increase the risk of developing thirteen types of cancer, including endometrial, breast, colorectal, liver, gallbladder, pancreas, and kidney. Obesity is responsible for about 4 to 8 percent of all cancers in the United States and is second only to tobacco use as a modifiable risk factor. Obesity prevents the immune system from functioning optimally, resulting in increased inflammation, insulin resistance, increased risk of diabetes, and overproduction of hormones and growth factors, all of which promote or fuel cancer development.

Excess body fat also makes it harder to screen for some cancers because getting clear images tends to require longer exposure to radiation, and some imaging equipment does not accommodate people over a certain size. Obesity is not exactly a lifestyle choice for many. It can be the result of low activity and bad nutrition choices, but it is also, more often, a larger metabolic issue. The bottom line in this context is that although obesity is one of the biggest risk factors for cancer, it is still one that can be modified.

Physical inactivity and sedentary lifestyles are also features of the Western lifestyle. These terms are not interchangeable. Being physically inactive means not meeting a recommended amount of physical activity. Being sedentary means spending extended amounts of time sitting or lying down while awake. The fact that many people have desk jobs nowadays means being sedentary is literally an occupational hazard, and screen time, which is such a big part of modern life, extends long after the workday.

Most Americans spend an average of 6.5 to 8 hours a day sitting down, according to the Centers for Disease Control and Prevention (CDC). A sedentary lifestyle has also been linked with cardiovascular risks and musculoskeletal issues. It is associated with insulin resistance and impaired glucose metabolism, it is a key factor in obesity, and it has been linked to mental health issues. Being physically active outside the workday is a big help, but the risk lies in those consecutive hours of prolonged sitting. Even people who exercise every day are at an elevated risk of cancer if they are sedentary the rest of the time. Being both sedentary and physically inactive is associated with the highest risk of cancer.

Alcohol consumption is linked to seven cancers, including oral, colorectal, liver, and breast. Alcohol converts to acetaldehyde in the body, which can damage DNA. Drinking and smoking together raises the risk of oral and esophageal cancers many times more than either of them alone, because alcohol acts as a solvent which helps harmful chemicals penetrate the tissues. It also interferes with the cells' natural repair processes and can prevent desirable nutrients like folate from being absorbed into the body properly. Heavy or binge drinking is a disastrous health risk on every level. For most cancers, the risk increases with increased alcohol consumption. But the risk of hormone receptor positive breast cancer especially, can increase even with small amounts of alcohol.

Sleep disruption, which includes insomnia, restless leg syndrome, and sleep apnea, is linked to an increased risk of breast, liver, colon, lung, pancreatic, and ovarian cancer. Circadian rhythm sleep disorders occur when the body's natural sleep-wake cycle is disrupted. Sleep deprivation is associated with a greater risk of colon polyps. And fragmented sleep triggers inflammation and can cause an imbalance of the appetite-regulating hormones, ghrelin and leptin, which are all related to obesity.

Poor sleep often leads to other high-risk behaviors as well. When people are sleep-deprived, they are more likely to eat high-carbohydrate and high-sugar foods and use tobacco and alcohol. And alcohol use interferes with deep sleep. According to the National Heart, Lung, and Blood Institute (NHLBI), 50–70 million people have ongoing sleep disorders, and in 2024, the National Council on Aging (NCOA) reported that more than a third of Americans are getting less than seven hours of sleep in a 24-hour period. And yet prioritizing sleep is free, and sleep disorders are usually readily treatable.

Melatonin is the hormone that regulates the circadian rhythm, which is the body's internal clock. The brain produces it in response to darkness and decreases production when it is light. Artificial light upsets this production leading to circadian rhythm disruption. The blue light emitted from LED bulbs, smartphones, desktop or laptop computers, tablets, or televisions can also suppress the production of melatonin. This negatively impacts immune function and hormone production, hinders cellular repair mechanisms, and increases oxidative stress and insulin resistance.

Melatonin also has an antioxidant and anti-inflammatory effect, which gives it anti-cancer properties, so interrupted melatonin production and circadian disruption have a compounded negative effect. Circadian disruption is common in shift work where people work in artificial light all night. As a result, the World Health Organization's International Agency for Research on Cancer (IARC) has classified shift work involving circadian disruption as probably carcinogenic to humans.

High-risk sexual behavior, which includes unprotected sex, unprotected oral sex, and multiple partners, is a lifestyle choice that is associated with the kinds of infections that can lead to cancer. The Epstein-Barr virus (EBV), Hepatitis B (HBV), Hepatitis C (HCV), the human herpesvirus 8 (HHV-8, also called Kaposi sarcoma-associated herpesvirus), the human immunodeficiency virus (HIV), and the human papillomavirus (HPV), can all be transmitted in body fluids through sexual contact. These viral infections increase the risk of cervical, vaginal, vulvar, penile, throat, anal, and liver cancer, among others. Although there are other ways to contract these infections, practicing safe sex is an obvious way to decrease the overall risk.

Stress is a lifestyle risk factor that is not always avoidable, but it can and should be managed. Studies are mixed when it comes to correlating stress to particular cancers, but a 2023 review of existing analyses found some evidence that psychological stress, stressful life events, depression, and anxiety can be linked to cancer incidence and mortality. Stress is strongly associated with other cancer risk factors like tobacco and alcohol use because it tends to lead to unhealthy behaviors and coping mechanisms. It also promotes cancer growth and spread because stress suppresses the immune system, triggers chronic inflammation and hormonal imbalance, increases blood pressure, and causes sleep disruption. All of these can result in long-term chemical changes in the body. Findings also suggest a relationship between stress and poor cancer outcomes.

Occupational exposure to certain chemicals is associated with certain cancers which are usually the result of a prolonged or extreme exposure not experienced by people outside that environment. Occupations with the highest cancer risk include pilots and air crews, firefighters, construction workers, agricultural workers, shift workers, people who work in rubber manufacturing, nail salon workers, mechanics, and miners.

And while changing jobs or professions is not always an option, cancers that occur because of workplace exposure are preventable if the exposure can be mitigated. Some measures require changes in behavior like getting up and moving more frequently, being assiduous about using personal protective equipment, or trying to stabilize a shift work schedule.

14. Which cancers can be hereditary?

Most cancers are "sporadic," caused by random mutations, sometimes but not always precipitated by lifestyle or environmental factors. Only a small percentage of cancers are caused by the kind of genetic mutations that can be inherited. According to the National Cancer Institute (NCI), between 5 and 10 percent of all cancers are hereditary.

Inherited cancer genes are the result of germline mutations, which means an individual has inherited an altered gene from one or both parents. This cancer-initiating gene, which is most commonly a tumor suppressor gene, is already copied into every cell of the body. Although the risk of cancer is greatly increased with a hereditary mutation, many additional mutations still need to occur for cancer to eventually develop. The hereditary mutation essentially starts the process one step further along. It may or may not happen, but it is more likely to happen than if the mutation were absent.

Many inherited mutations are associated with specific cancer syndromes. Hereditary cancer syndromes cause certain patterns of cancer to appear within the same family. Although the terms "hereditary risk" and "family history" may be used interchangeably, hereditary risk implies a known genetic link. A family history of cancer can occur due to factors like a shared environment, exposure, lifestyle habits, or a combination of genetic markers.

Some mutations are autosomal dominant, meaning that if a parent has the gene, each of his or her children has a 50 percent chance of inheriting it. Autosomal recessive cancer mutations are mutations that must be inherited from both parents for there to be a predisposition for cancer. People with one copy of the mutation are carriers, and if both parents are carriers each child has a 25 percent chance of inheriting the mutation.

Sometimes the inherited mutation is epigenetic, a change in gene expression rather than a mutation. When there is an epigenetic modification, the DNA sequence remains intact but certain genes are switched on or off. These changes are associated with some cancers, diabetes, autoimmune diseases, and mental disorders. This gene activation, or deactivation, remains in daughter cells as they multiply, and can be passed down from parent to child. Epigenetic changes are part of normal development, cellular differentiation, and aging, but can be also caused by environmental exposure, drugs or pharmaceuticals, or diet.

The two most common hereditary syndromes are hereditary breast and ovarian cancer syndrome (HBOC), and Lynch Syndrome. HBOC is associated with a mutation in the BRCA1 and BRCA2 genes. Women with the BRCA1 mutation have a 55 to 72 percent lifetime risk of developing breast cancer, compared to a 13 percent lifetime risk for the general population. Breast cancer associated with BRCA1 is likely to be the more aggressive triple-negative breast cancer, and the mutation also increases the risk of ovarian and pancreatic cancers. Men with the mutation are at a slightly higher risk of developing prostate cancer.

Women with the BRCA2 mutation have a 45 to 69 percent lifetime risk of developing breast cancer, and the cancer linked to this mutation is more likely to be hormone receptor positive breast cancer. It is also associated with an increased risk of ovarian and pancreatic cancers, as well as melanoma. Men with the BRCA2 mutation have a significantly higher risk of developing male breast cancer, even though the likelihood is still very low. But they also face an increased risk of developing other cancers including prostate, pancreatic, and colon.

Lynch syndrome is caused by a mutation in one of five genes that can increase the risk of many cancers, especially earlier in life. It is particularly associated with colorectal and endometrial cancer. The lifetime risk of developing colorectal cancer for the general population is about 5 percent, but it jumps to a lifetime risk of between 40 and 80 percent for people with this genetic condition. Genetic testing for Lynch syndrome is generally recommended for people with a family history of early cancer diagnoses, or an immediate relative who has been diagnosed with Lynch syndrome.

Some other hereditary cancer syndromes include hereditary retinoblastoma, an eye cancer that mainly affects children, and familial adenomatous polyposis, a condition which causes polyps to grow in the intestinal tract and increases the risk of colorectal cancers. Inherited genes are also associated with specific types of bone, stomach, thyroid, and testicular cancers, as well as some types of leukemia and lymphoma.

A thorough personal and medical history is required to assess the risk of an inherited genetic mutation. Some indications of genetic risk might include getting a cancer diagnosis at an early age, any history of a rare cancer, or cancer on both sides of a paired organ like kidneys or breasts. Family history is collected to find out if multiple people in the same family are being diagnosed with the same or related cancers, highlighting the importance of maintaining a family medical history. This information can help a medical professional decide whether genetic testing is appropriate.

Germline genetic testing looks for changes in the DNA inherited from your parents. Somatic genetic testing looks at genetic mutations that may have occurred in the body after you were born. Some tests look for one specific gene, whereas genetic panels will show all or groups of genes.

Genetic testing often involves speaking with a genetic counselor, a professional qualified to explain and advise on what can sometimes be very unsettling medical information. Knowing if you have a mutation that increases your chances of developing cancer can help you prioritize your risk management. It might initiate some lifestyle changes and encourage the necessary screening for early detection. In some cases, knowing in advance there is an elevated risk could prompt some people to take preemptive medication or action, such as banking sperm or eggs. In some cases, people even consider having prophylactic, or preventive, surgery to remove the organ at risk. Knowing about cancer-related mutations would also alert family members to their own potential risk and allow them to take action as well.

While getting genetic testing can provide valuable information, it often raises new questions. Grappling with the results can be stressful, especially when outcomes are uncertain. Some people may fixate on the findings or become overly anxious. These challenges are even more pronounced with direct-to-consumer genetic tests, which may lack the professional support needed for proper interpretation. Without guidance, individuals might make rash decisions based on incomplete or misunderstood results. A positive result simply means the mutation is present, but it does not guarantee cancer will develop. A negative result means the mutation is absent, but it does not eliminate the general risk of cancer that exists for everyone. (See Question 4—What role does mutation play in cancer development?)

15. Are you more likely to get cancer again if you have had it before?

Compared to people who have never had cancer before, cancer survivors do have an increased risk of developing another cancer, even after surviving the first one. In some cases, residual dormant cancer cells in the body, missed by the initial treatment, reemerge and grow after months or years. This is a metastatic recurrence, or a secondary cancer, meaning it is the same type as the original cancer. In other cases, a cancer survivor might develop an unrelated, or new kind of cancer. This is called a second cancer or second primary cancer. Leukemias, lymphomas, and sarcomas are the most common second cancers, along with breast, lung, and thyroid.

According to the National Cancer Institute (NCI), one in five people diagnosed with cancer has had cancer before. Part of the elevated risk is simply associated with the fact that cancer survivors now live longer, and the chance of getting any cancer increases with age. But the odds of developing a second cancer also vary a great deal depending on what the primary cancer was, what the treatment was, and the patient's age at diagnosis. For instance, the most common second cancer in survivors of melanoma is another skin cancer. The most common second cancer in breast cancer survivors is another breast cancer.

Sometimes cancer is a random occurrence, and although fairly unlikely, it is possible that a second cancer might be equally random. The second cancer might be completely unrelated to the first. Sometimes, cancer survivors get a second cancer for the same reasons they had it before. The same risk factors may still exist. Unhealthy lifestyle habits and environmental or occupational exposures might lead to cancer again, but in a different place. Reducing the chances of a second cancer involves changing the risk factors that might have precipitated the first.

Someone might develop a second cancer because they are genetically predisposed to getting the disease, such as having inherited mutations that make any kind of cancer more likely. Or they have an inherited cancer syndrome, which is a mutation-specific pattern of cancers seen within families and which often involves developing two or more types of cancer. Some individuals with certain hereditary disorders have increased sensitivity to the effects of radiation and could be at a higher risk after their initial cancer treatments.

Cancer treatment itself increases risk because several therapies that cancer patients receive are themselves potentially carcinogenic. Chemotherapy, radiation, and bone marrow transplants are all linked with specific types of second cancers. Some chemotherapy drugs are associated with increased risk of acute myeloid leukemia. The kind of radiation that destroys cancer cells can also damage the DNA of healthy cells. The stronger the radiation, the higher the risk. Radiation is associated with second cancers like leukemia, breast, and thyroid cancer. Children who were treated for Hodgkin lymphoma with chest radiation are at an especially high risk for developing breast cancer, for example. Having a weakened immune system, either from previous disease or immunosuppression from cancer treatment, also increases risk.

Cancer treatment is often about weighing risks and benefits, but the benefits usually outweigh the small risk of a second cancer, and many treatments are now more carefully targeted and less likely to cause the kind of damage they used to. Given how much impact the fear of cancer recurrence can have on a cancer survivor, it is important for them to keep monitoring with screenings and blood tests. (See Question 43—What happens if the treatment fails or the cancer comes back?)

16. How can you lower your risk of getting cancer?

Cancer risk is generally linked to things that are beyond the control of an individual or a health care system, like age, gender, ethnicity, genetic background, family history, medical history, place of origin, and past exposures. But almost half of all cancer deaths worldwide are attributed to modifiable risk factors. Modifiable, because they involve behaviors and habits. Ultimately, this means it is possible to lower your risk of getting cancer. The problem with effective cancer prevention is that the disease is not an immediate consequence of risky behavior, so there seems to be little urgency. And because risk varies among individuals for reasons we still do not fully understand, people, especially young people, assume it will never happen to them.

There is a growing interest in preventive and integrative approaches to health, full of terms like biohacking (using science and self-experimentation to improve overall health) and holistic health (identifying and addressing root causes and treating the whole person). These concepts are relevant to what we are coming to know about cancer prevention, and can inform what you can do, today, to lower your risk of getting cancer.

Metabolic health might be one of the most important things you could address in lowering the risk of cancer. Any pamphlet, book, or webpage dedicated to chronic or age-related illness, and the American Cancer Society (ACS) is no exception, will have the same list of recommendations that all basically consist of improving metabolic health. Metabolism is the foundation of all the processes of the body which break down food and use energy. Metabolic health refers to the optimal functioning of the body. Medically, it means having healthy levels of blood sugar, triglycerides, high-density lipoprotein cholesterol (HDL), blood pressure that falls within a normal range, and healthy waist circumference, all without the use of medications.

Being metabolically unhealthy is associated with heart disease, diabetes, strokes, liver and kidney diseases, neurodegenerative diseases like Alzheimer's and Parkinson's, and cancer. Metabolic risk factors contribute to nearly one-fifth of all cancer deaths in men and one fourth of all cancer deaths in women. Improving metabolic health involves a healthy diet, physical activity, healthy weight, good sleep, stress management, and reducing chronic inflammation.

A healthy diet is what the ACS recommends for lowering the risk of cancer. This includes a variety of nutritious and whole foods like fruits, vegetables, whole grains, and lean meats; and limits (or eliminates) red and processed meats, sugar sweetened beverages, highly processed foods, and refined grain products. The key is variety and moderation.

Eating a variety of foods together is more beneficial than any one food on its own. Nutrient diversity is also better for the microbiome, the bacteria in your gut that break down carbohydrates and help synthesize essential vitamins. A healthy microbiome is linked to better digestion and a stronger immune system.

Whole and healthy foods are also better at balancing blood sugar levels in the bloodstream. The body is designed to use nutrients to function and heal, and it uses these nutrients more efficiently when it gets them from whole healthy food. People have different philosophies about food, and they may tolerate or digest foods differently, so a balanced diet of whole, healthy foods will probably look slightly different for everyone.

Dietary habits can impact cancer risk especially by affecting the lining of the large bowel. Fried, fast, and fatty foods, and foods high in refined carbohydrates and sugars increase the risk of polyps and chronic inflammatory bowel disease. The Food and Drug Administration (FDA) does not currently have an official classification for processed versus ultra-processed foods, but generally, processed foods are defined as having been changed from their natural whole state to make them convenient or prolong their shelf life. This kind of processing includes cutting, heating, canning, and dehydrating. Processed foods include things like frozen vegetables, cheese, or tofu. Ultra-processed foods have undergone industrial processes and contain chemical additives and preservatives. These foods can often be highly altered, high in calories, sugars, fats, or salt, and low in fiber, protein, vitamins, and minerals. They can interfere with the body's satiety, or natural hunger signals, and cause spikes in blood sugar levels, leading to insulin resistance and chronic inflammation over time.

A diet rich in fruits and vegetables, which contain cancer fighting phytochemicals and antioxidants, whole grains, and lean proteins such as legumes, fish, and chicken, is associated with better metabolic health. Some foods, including cruciferous vegetables, fatty fish, berries, nuts, and probiotic foods like yogurt and kimchi, also fight inflammation. And while taking supplements might be helpful, it is useful to remember that they should "supplement" healthy foods, not replace them.

The Mediterranean diet is recommended by several organizations like the American Heart Association and the American Institute for Cancer Research. Studies suggest that it is associated with reduced risk of overall cancer mortality. It is a diet routinely recommended by doctors and nutritionists because its foundation consists of whole, mostly unprocessed foods, like whole grains, beans, and nuts, an infinite variety of fruits and vegetables, moderate amounts of lean proteins, eggs, and dairy products, and limited red meats and sweet treats. It heavily features heart-healthy olive oil and even includes the occasional glass of wine. It also lends itself easily to being vegetarian or vegan. People who follow a Mediterranean diet tend to live longer and have a lower risk of frailty, lower rates of depression, and report higher levels of well-being and satisfaction.

Physical activity is recommended to lower the risk of many diseases. The ACS recommends 150 to 300 minutes of moderate intensity exercise, or 75 to 150 minutes of vigorous intensity exercise every week. Children and teens should get at least an hour of activity each day. Moderately intense activity might include walking, dancing, or yoga, or a sport like golf or badminton. Vigorous intensity might include running, swimming, basketball, or tennis. Productive physical activities at home or in the workplace, like gardening, cleaning, or building are also good for you. Aerobic exercise, strength, and resistance training to build muscle mass, and short bursts of intense exercise like high-intensity interval training (HIIT), improve cardiovascular health and insulin sensitivity, boost the immune system, regulate hormones, reduce inflammation, and improve metabolism.

A 2016 *Journal of the American Medical Association* meta-analysis showed high levels of physical activity were linked to a 7 percent lower risk of cancer. Another study in the same publication showed physical activity was associated with lower risks of cancer regardless of other risk factors like body size or smoking history. But being physically active does not just imply working out. It is also especially important to avoid sitting all day. Those consecutive hours at a desk or on the couch are a problem even for people who do exercise. It might feel forced or artificial to make time to move, but in fact it is the sedentary lifestyle that is artificial. Our bodies are designed to move, and they serve us best when we do. Good metabolic health depends on finding ways to break up the hours of immobility, like taking a break to stand, stretch or walk, using a standing desk, or pacing during phone calls.

Healthy body weight is one of many markers of metabolic health. Obesity is associated with the increased risk of thirteen types of cancer. But body weight is not the only, or even the best predictor of metabolic health. In fact, the number on the scale is not necessarily the number you should worry about. It is more important to focus on body composition. A waist circumference of more than 35 inches for women, and 40 inches for men, is a better predictor for metabolic disease risk. Visceral fat, or fat that is carried around the middle, is especially associated with diabetes and cancer risk.

Obesity is measured using the body mass index (BMI) which is calculated by dividing a person's weight in pounds by their height in inches squared and multiplying by 703. A BMI of 25.0 to 29.9 is considered overweight and a BMI of 30.0 and above is considered obese. BMI is not the most accurate tool but can be used as one of many metrics for health. Being overweight young is an even greater risk factor than gaining weight later in life, so disease prevention should critically include encouraging and modeling healthy behaviors for children.

Important markers for metabolic health also include blood pressure, blood glucose, triglyceride, and cholesterol levels. These levels tend to increase or decrease alongside weight gain and weight loss. So ultimately, achieving a healthy weight could also bring other metabolic health markers to healthy levels. It might even take the pressure off losing weight to focus on the other health markers first. Excess weight is linked to so many health concerns that the smallest changes in the right direction can make a difference. Telling people to lose weight is a crude oversimplification of what may be a complex metabolic issue, but telling them their weight is not a problem is a dangerous disservice.

Sleep is an untapped competitive advantage. When people are well rested, they make better decisions, have better judgment, are more cognitively stable and alert, and have faster reactions. Adequate sleep also helps regulate immune responses. Poor sleep has been linked to insulin resistance, weight gain, and hormonal imbalance, all of which are cancer risk factors. The ideal number of recommended hours of sleep can vary, but the American Academy of Sleep Medicine recommends that adults get seven or more hours of sleep per night, noting there is no upper limit on that number, because sleeping more than nine hours per night regularly may still be appropriate for young adults or people who are ill or recovering from sleep debt.

Having a good sleep routine, also known as sleep hygiene, involves taking on certain habits that will improve your sleep quality. The sleeping environment should be pleasant, quiet, dark, and quite cool. A wind-down routine that includes reading or meditating can calm a racing mind. Avoiding stimulants like caffeine, tobacco, and alcohol, heavy meals, and exercise right before bed is also helpful.

Television, phone, computer, and tablet screens are huge culprits in causing poor sleep because the blue light they emit suppresses melatonin production. Whether flashing notifications make you feel like you are in constant response mode, or whether doom scrolling on social media for hours cuts into your sleep time, it is best to put devices away while winding down for bed. Going to bed and waking up at the same times each day seems to be protective for metabolic health as well, because a consistent sleep schedule supports the body's natural circadian rhythm. If sleep is a challenge, it is a good idea to get tested for sleep apnea. Untreated sleep apnea is associated with cardiovascular issues and high blood pressure. Sleep should not be a negotiable part of your schedule, and the best part is that it is free, healthy, and safe.

Stress has been called the silent killer. Acute stress, the short-term physiological and psychological reaction to a specific event, is normal and even beneficial in a crisis. But chronic stress, which is long-term, persistent, and overwhelming, can lead to immune disorders, hormonal imbalances, weight gain, and chronic inflammation. It disrupts sleep and leads to unhealthy coping behaviors like smoking or poor diet, which are also cancer risk factors. Managing stress can involve psychological intervention or drugs. But the strategies outlined here, like exercise and diet, also have a compound benefit on stress reduction. Things like meditation, yoga, and breath work are useful in calming a nervous system in distress.

In 2023, the Department of Health and Human Services published an advisory about social media and youth mental health. Many studies show that constant connectivity, social media, and screen time have been associated with obesity, physical inactivity, depression, anxiety, and mood disorders. A digital detox, refraining from using electronic devices and social media for a while, has become popular as people become more aware of the mental health impact of technology. It is an easy way to reduce stress, improve focus, and it encourages people to engage with one another in person.

In fact, the Centers for Disease Control and Prevention (CDC) reports that social connection and personal relationships have a positive effect on physical and mental health. Social connection includes in-person as well as online interactions, as long as they are sustaining meaningful relationships. People with high-quality relationships live longer, have better sleep, healthier habits, less anxiety, and a lower risk of chronic diseases and dementia. Staying connected with friends, family, and community is part of the human experience and our social animal brains crave it.

Reducing inflammation may be one of the best ways of lowering the risk of cancer. Like stress, inflammation can be acute or chronic. Acute inflammation is the immune system's normal, short-term, response to infection or injury. Chronic inflammation is inflammation that does not go away, and which continues even when it is unnecessary. This is the kind of inflammation that promotes cancer development. Most strategies to lower cancer risk work because they help to limit the causes of chronic inflammation, like a healthy diet and exercise. Smoking, alcohol, obesity, sleep deprivation, and stress all promote chronic inflammation. Some health conditions, medications, toxins, and infections can also activate this inflammatory response. It may take the help of a medical professional to tease out its causes so it can be treated. Improving immune function does more than lower chronic inflammation, an efficient and healthy immune system cleans up cellular waste and debris, and recognizes and destroys abnormal cells.

Tobacco is on every list of health risks. According to the CDC, smoking is the leading cause of preventable disease, disability, and death in the United States.

The best thing someone can do to lower their risk of getting cancer, and a great many other diseases, is to quit smoking, or never start. The risk of developing lung cancer in a current pack a day smoker for forty years is approximately twenty times higher than the risk of someone who has never smoked. And smoking does not only reduce lifespan, but it also reduces health span, or years of healthy living. When people quit smoking, their risk falls significantly compared to people who have continued to smoke, so it is never too late. But it is difficult. Smokers are not undisciplined, they have a very powerful physical and psychological addiction, and quitting any addiction is very hard. Sometimes quitting may seem impossible or even undesirable. But even just reducing the overall exposure to harmful chemicals, and reducing cancer risk in other ways, through exercise and diet, may help. Nicotine replacement therapies and support groups are easy to find. Every little bit counts, even if the damage is already done.

Alcohol is a risk factor associated with overlapping risks, which means that people who drink often practice other high-risk behaviors like smoking, as well. For some people, alcohol is a cultural part of social occasions and celebrations, it helps them feel more socially engaged and relaxed, it is associated with conviviality and hospitality, even ceremony. There is some evidence, as published in a 2024 report from the National Academies of Sciences, Engineering, and Medicine, that very moderate consumption of alcohol is associated with lower mortality rates. But the reality is that even small amounts of alcohol can stress the body to some degree, and excessive alcohol consumption is implicated in many mental and physical health problems.

The bottom line for cancer risk is that alcohol can cause insulin resistance, hormonal imbalance, liver damage, and chronic inflammation. It is addictive and toxic. People who want to drink should drink moderately and if they cannot drink moderately, they should not drink at all. Moderate consumption is defined as one standard drink per day for women and two for men. Heavy drinking is defined as more than three drinks per day for women and four for men.

The kind of drinking that should be encouraged is water for hydration. The National Council on Aging reports that 75 percent of Americans are chronically dehydrated, yet proper hydration is essential for metabolism and reducing inflammation. Drinking plenty of water throughout the day supports digestion and nutrient absorption. Hydrated organs and cells function better and flush toxins more efficiently.

Sun protection is crucial in avoiding sunburn. Being prone to or having a history of bad sunburn increases the risk of skin cancer, but many people are not aware that a suntan is still sun damage, and exposure is cumulative. The extra melanin in tanned or darker skin only provides a sun protection factor (SPF) of about 2 to 10. The best way to prevent skin cancer is to avoid getting sunburned.

A good way to gauge risk is to monitor the ultraviolet (UV) index, which is a daily forecast for UV radiation. A UV index of 1 to 2 is low, over 8 is very high to extreme. The UV index is usually highest between 11:00 AM and 3:00 PM, so it helps to plan outdoor activities for mornings and evenings.

During high UV index times, meaning an index of 3 and up, you should apply a broad-spectrum, water-resistant sunscreen with a sun protection factor (SPF) of 30 or higher to skin that is not covered. Try to stay in the shade, wear protective clothing or clothing with an ultraviolet protection factor (UPF) number on the label, and wear a hat and sunglasses.

To get the SPF protection indicated on the sunscreen's label, make sure you use what the American Academy of Dermatology Association recommends; one ounce, or a shot glass-full, to cover the whole body, or a nickel sized blob to cover the face. When used incorrectly, sunscreen may give a false sense of protection, so it is essential to use the right amount and reapply it as directed.

People should also be aware that UV rays are stronger at high altitudes and closer to the equator, that snow, sand, and water reflect UV radiation and can double exposure, and that it can still penetrate light cloud cover. Certain things may make you more sensitive to UV radiation, such as medications like antibiotics and cholesterol-lowering drugs, or using certain skin care products that contain retinoids and acids.

Most car and building windows block UVB radiation, which is the shorter wavelength radiation most likely to cause sunburn, but they do not block UVA, which is the longer wavelength radiation associated with long-term skin damage. It is critical to take special care that children avoid sunburn since sunburn during childhood is one of the most significant risks of future skin cancer. And although melanoma of the eye is extremely rare, polarized sunglasses that offer 100 percent UV protection can protect the eyes from sun damage and prevent cataracts and macular degeneration.

The evidence that tanning beds increase the risk of developing melanoma and other skin cancers is so strong that the FDA requires warning labels on indoor tanning equipment. It is safest to avoid them altogether because the bottom line is that there is no such thing as a healthy tan, only skin damage. Self-tanning sprays or lotions are a better option, and new products no longer leave you looking like an orange popsicle.

Keep in mind there are many health benefits to spending time outside in green spaces, including getting sunlight. Sunlight is really incredibly good for humans, it helps the body produce vitamin D, it releases serotonin and improves mental health, it helps to prevent seasonal affective disorder (SAD), and regulates sleep cycles. Do not avoid sunshine, avoid sunburn. Get outside as much as you can and protect yourself as much as you need to.

Risky behavior can increase cancer risk. People associate risky behavior with sex, drugs, and rock'n'roll. The good news is that rock'n'roll is not a risk factor for cancer. But high-risk sex and substance abuse are. Contracting a viral infection like human papillomavirus (HPV) or human immunodeficiency virus (HIV) through unprotected sex or sharing needles can result in certain cancers down the road. Safe sex practices include communicating with your partner about sexual health and history, limiting partners, using physical barriers like condoms, and staying current on checkups for sexual health, which includes getting tested and treated for sexually transmitted infections. Some studies also indicate that men with fewer sexual partners, older age at first intercourse, and moderately frequent ejaculations, had a significantly decreased risk of prostate cancer.

Substance use and abuse are also cancer risks, depending on the substance and how it is taken. Smoking, snorting, or huffing anything will damage airways and lungs and lead to chronic inflammation. Anabolic steroids disrupt normal hormone production. Illicit drugs can be toxic on their own but become highly carcinogenic if they are cut or laced with other chemicals.

Staying informed and getting medical care are important ways to lower cancer risk. These will include getting regular checkups and preventive care, getting vaccines against infections like HPV, which can result in cancer, and receiving important guidance, like nutrition advice or smoking cessation. Seeing a medical professional regularly will also help you assess risk and stay current on cancer screenings, which are vital because if you cannot prevent cancer, your best chance is to catch it as early as possible. Knowing your family history can make a difference as to which screenings you should have, or how early you have them. And it is always worth asking about new symptoms, strange moles, or odd lumps. If any symptoms have lasted longer than a week or two, they should not be dismissed. Knowing for sure is better than any awkwardness or embarrassment you might feel about asking.

As with anything in life, being aware and staying informed is at least empowering, and at best, lifesaving. Following the latest headlines about research and tracking cancer awareness and prevention programs helps people notice issues earlier and communicate them better to a doctor. Advocating for your health starts with education. Is it possible that having checked every single box in cancer prevention, someone might still get cancer? Of course, risk is probability. But optimizing health can also massively improve their chances of beating cancer if they do get it. A healthy body will put up a harder fight.

Avoiding environmental or occupational exposure to possible carcinogens might be harder to address. Depending on when and where a structure was built, it may be important to talk to a home inspector or real estate agent about testing for things like asbestos or radon. It might be necessary to hire professionals to safely remove them or install ventilation, detectors, or countermeasures. Both the ACS and the Environmental Protection Agency (EPA) offer guidelines and suggestions. Air pollution is also harder to avoid, but being aware of the air quality index (AQI) can inform when and how much time you should spend outside. Indoors, using filters and air purifiers can reduce dangerous particles.

Cancer risk involves overlapping factors which are multiplicative. This means one risk factor increases the chance of having other risk factors. If you are physically inactive, there is a good chance that you might be overweight. If you have a high-stress lifestyle there is a good chance that you are eating a poor diet, drinking alcohol, or smoking tobacco. And each of these risk factors multiplies the chances of developing cancer. But it is crucial to recognize that this process works in reverse as well. If you start being physically active you are more likely to start doing other healthy things like sleeping better, being more social, going outside, and experiencing less stress. One healthy habit could start a cascade of other healthy habits. Do not believe that small changes are inconsequential.

17. Which cancers are preventable?

Cancer is not 100 percent preventable. But over 40 percent of cancers worldwide are attributed to risk factors that can be changed. Measures that control or curb risky behaviors and exposures can have a quantifiable effect on cancer incidence. Preventing cancer would have a massive impact on individuals as well as health care systems. On an economic level, prevention is the most cost-effective strategy in lowering the burden of cancer. On a personal level, prevention is always better than intervention.

Cervical cancer is the most preventable cancer. The World Health Organization (WHO) estimates that 99 percent of cervical cancer cases are caused by a human papillomavirus (HPV) infection. This infection can be easily screened for using Pap tests and/or HPV tests, and it can be prevented by getting the HPV vaccine which is 97 percent effective. The vaccine is most effective if given to children (male and female) age eleven to twelve so they can be fully protected before they become sexually active, but it is also available to people up to the age of forty-five. Vaccination is critical in preventing more than cervical cancer. The National Cancer Institute (NCI) estimates that HPV also causes over 90 percent of anal cancer, 70 percent of throat cancer, 63 percent of penile cancer, 75 percent of vaginal cancer, and 69 percent of vulvar cancer. It is important to raise awareness of the fact that the risks of having unprotected vaginal, anal, and oral sex include sexually transmitted infections that can result in cancer.

Given a vaccine and effective early detection, why is the NCI projecting almost 14,000 new cases in 2024? There are still geographical and financial barriers to getting vaccines, screenings, and treatment. In addition, certain demographic groups do not realize they are at risk. Anyone with a history of abnormal results should keep screening even if they are over the recommended age of sixty-five. Transgender men who have a cervix can also be at risk for cervical cancer and should stay current with their preventive care.

Lung cancer (including tracheal and bronchus) is the leading cause of cancer-related deaths worldwide. It can be linked to several risk factors, but the most important is cigarette smoking. The World Health Organization (WHO) reports that smoking causes 1.2 million lung cancer deaths each year and estimates that 85 percent of all cases of lung cancer are related to smoking. Therefore, the most significant way to prevent lung cancer is to persuade people to quit smoking or never start.

Secondhand smoke, or passive smoke, is also a significant risk factor for lung cancer and should be avoided, especially in enclosed areas like cars, or bars and restaurants. Public health campaigns have had an impact on cigarette smoking in the United States. Smoking has been slowly declining since the 1970s and as a result, lung cancer incidence has followed by slowly declining since the 1990s. At a policy level, lung cancer can also be prevented by reducing residential and occupational exposure to radon gas, and other environmental carcinogens, as well as addressing air pollution levels.

Oral, throat, and esophageal cancers are often associated with tobacco and alcohol because these substances are in direct contact with the tissues that line the mouth and throat. Some of these cancers can be prevented by limiting or avoiding tobacco and alcohol, having good oral hygiene, and managing chronic reflux issues.

Skin cancer is the most common cancer in the United States, with over 6 million people diagnosed every year, according to the Centers for Disease Control and Prevention (CDC). Because over 95 percent of skin cancers, mostly squamous and basal cell carcinomas, are caused by UV exposure, they are a very preventable type of cancer. Melanoma only accounts for about 1 percent of skin cancers, but it is by far the deadliest form because of its aggressive ability to spread. Prevention consists of helping people become aware of risk factors like having fair skin, blond or red hair, freckles, or moles, which makes them more likely to get sunburned. But awareness should also be raised among people with deeper skin tones because they are also at risk. Although people of color are less prone to getting any kind of skin cancer, if they are diagnosed with melanoma, they are statistically more likely to die from it. This is because it is generally diagnosed at a much later, more advanced, stage. People with deeper skin tones delay getting medical care because the risk is perceived to be low. And because some melanomas are harder to identify on darker skin, or appear in unexpected places such as the palms, soles of feet, or under finger and toenails, they can be overlooked.

Preventing skin cancer means everyone should protect their skin from prolonged or intense sun exposure by covering it up and using a broad-spectrum water-resistant sunscreen. Children especially should be protected from UV overexposure because serious burns sustained in childhood are a risk factor for skin cancer later in life.

People should also be aware of the dangers of tanning beds, as tanning beds or booths emit ten to fifteen times more UV rays than the sun. According to the American Academy of Dermatology, indoor tanning increases the risk of squamous cell carcinoma by 58 percent and basal cell carcinoma by 24 percent. In addition, everyone should simply be checking their skin on a regular basis for bumps or sores that do not heal, or moles that have changed size, color, or shape, because even if skin cancer cannot be prevented, it can probably be cured if caught early.

Colorectal cancer risk is associated with a wide range of risk factors. But a little over half of colorectal cancer deaths are attributed to risk factors that are modifiable. Managing body weight, physical activity, and diet can reduce risk. This is the area of the body where food is digested and nutrients are absorbed so it is no surprise that avoiding things that cause chronic inflammation, like red and processed meats and alcohol, will help. Colorectal cancer can also be prevented with regular colonoscopy screenings to find and remove intestinal polyps before they develop into cancer. A 2019 study in the *Journal of the American Medical Association* found that regular colonoscopies reduced the risk of developing colorectal cancer by 46 percent.

Liver cancer can be caused by infections in the liver, and in fact, the leading cause of liver cancer in the United States is hepatitis. Hepatitis B (HBV) is now less common in the United States because there is routine vaccination against it, and Hepatitis C (HCV) can be treated with an antiviral. These infections are transmitted through blood, sexual contact, or sharing needles. Liver cancer is also associated with cirrhosis, a chronic and irreversible liver disease. Because the liver plays a key role in digestion and blood filtration, it is exposed to many damaging and toxic substances. Liver cancer could be prevented by getting vaccinated for HBV, staying hydrated, managing any chronic liver disease early and assiduously, and cutting back on things like tobacco and alcohol.

Other more common cancers like bladder, kidney, pancreatic, and breast cancer are preventable to a varying degree. Regular screenings help to prevent disease because anything that risks developing into cancer can be found and removed. Some hereditary cancers might be prevented by getting genetic testing done and having prophylactic treatment. With most cancers, prevention begins with being as healthy as possible.

18. What are carcinogens?

Carcinogens are chemical, physical, or biological agents that promote the kinds of mutations or cell behaviors that result in cancer development. Carcinogens can be mutagens, meaning they can initiate mutations. But they can also indirectly stimulate cancer development by disrupting the cell cycle to stimulate cell growth or inhibit cell death. So, all mutagens are carcinogens, but not all carcinogens are mutagens.

Different carcinogens are linked to different cancers, but no single carcinogen can cause all cancers. Some are the byproducts of human activity, and some are naturally occurring. Some of these agents can be beneficial in small amounts but dangerous in large ones. Being exposed to a carcinogen does not automatically cause cancer, the risk often depends on the length and extent of the exposure, and the physical idiosyncrasies of the individual.

There are over 100 known carcinogens, some of which we are exposed to every day like the tiny amounts of arsenic in drinking water, or the pollution in the air we breathe. They can be chemicals, like asbestos, and benzene. Physical carcinogens include radiation like ultraviolet (UV) rays from the sun or ionizing radiation from radon gas or x-rays. And they can also be biological, like bacteria, parasites, or viruses.

Exposure to carcinogens can be environmental, meaning they are simply present all around us in the air and water. They can come from exposure to household items, pesticides, or industrial chemicals, or naturally occurring exposures like sunlight or infection. Some exposures are occupational or associated with specific workplaces like factories and other industrial sites, laboratories, and health care settings.

Some medical treatments are carcinogenic, including, ironically, chemotherapy and radiation. And finally, there is a broad variety of lifestyle factors that expose us to carcinogens, including tobacco and alcohol. In 2021, the National Toxicology Program (NTP) reported that there is "high confidence" that shift work is "probably carcinogenic to humans" based on studies that show a connection between cancer and sleep cycle disorders.

Agencies like the NTP and the Environmental Protection Agency (EPA) in the United States, and the International Agency for Research on Cancer (IARC), which is part of the World Health Organization (WHO), constantly assess research and generate lists of carcinogens. The IARC classifies these agents into four groups depending on the evidence of their cancer-causing potential:

Group 1: Carcinogenic to humans—these are known carcinogens like smoking, radiation, chronic Hepatitis B infection, and processed meats.

Group 2A: Probably carcinogenic to humans—There is some good evidence that these are carcinogens, but with a lower degree of confidence. This group includes high temperature frying, some insecticides, and lead compounds.

Group 2B: Possibly carcinogenic to humans—there is limited evidence these cause cancer in humans, although there might be some evidence they cause cancer in animals. So, more research is needed to know for sure about things on this list like engine exhaust, aspartame, and progestins.

Group 3: Not classifiable as to its carcinogenicity in humans—there is simply not enough evidence to say that these things, like caffeine, chlorinated water, or acetaminophen, have any link to cancer.

Similar systems are used by the NTP and EPA where the criteria are either "Known to be a Human Carcinogen" or "Reasonably Anticipated to be a Human Carcinogen." It is particularly important to note that these classifications are qualitative (is there a risk?) but not quantitative (what is the magnitude of the risk?). Classification does not assess the probability of causing cancer. It only assesses whether the potential to cause cancer exists, based on the evidence available.

For instance, IARC classifies tobacco in the same group as processed meat. This does not mean a hotdog is as deadly as a cigarette which contains at least seventy known carcinogens. It means both these things have the same level and quality of evidence to support their classification. These agencies review all the studies available, evaluate the quality of the evidence, and update their findings as the information is revised. The less evidence exists, the lower the agent's place in the ranking. Identifying something as a carcinogen is tricky. Something that is linked to cancer does not automatically mean it causes cancer.

Testing a carcinogen can be impossible in some cases, and real proof is hard to come by. The time between exposure and disease is unpredictable. In vitro studies and rodent models, though important in research, cannot conclusively show that a substance causes cancer in humans. It is unethical for scientists to expose people to a potential carcinogen to see if they get sick. And observational evidence collected through epidemiological studies is slow, expensive, and must allow for the fact that people have vast genetic differences, and do not live in a controlled environment. It is also common for studies to contradict each other. In essence, identifying something as carcinogenic is only based on trends correlated to exposure, strong association, and a high probability of causality. By the time an agent has been labeled a carcinogen, a fairly strong case has to be built to support its classification.

Criticisms leveled against these classifications are that different agencies sometimes publish contradictory reports, and that these reports often cause waves of media coverage that can be both inaccurate and fear mongering. Ultimately, the benefits are that this information is used by national health agencies to inform legislation, screening guidelines, and occupational safety standards worldwide. They hopefully encourage the development of safer alternatives, better regulatory standards, and better public health.

At this time, testing chemicals for their cancer-causing potential involves exposing mice and waiting to see if they develop cancer, a process which can take about two years. But research is ongoing into developing tests that could identify potential carcinogens by watching specialized human liver-like cells for the tell-tale signs of DNA damage.

There are many misconceptions about things which people believe cause cancer, such as cell phone use, power lines, microwaves, antiperspirants, soy products, underwired bras, and artificial sweeteners. Studies so far have failed to show a link between these things and cancer. At best, the information is inconclusive.

Although it is easy to correlate many of these things with cancer, correlation does not imply causation. Just because a statistical relationship exists between two variables does not mean one is causing the other. A classic example of spurious correlation is the rise of cheese consumption being closely related to the number of people who die by becoming entangled in their bed sheets. There is an indisputable correlation between the two, but one is clearly not the cause of the other.

Certain items have changed their manufacturing and are safer than they used to be, like Teflon, which used to contain PFOAs but no longer does. However, many people still believe it causes cancer. Some things are a question of dose and exposure. For example, x-rays are considered carcinogens, but the levels used in imaging tests are very low, lower than the average amount of background radiation people are exposed to every day.

So, are people worrying about the wrong things? Yes and no. It is possible that in the future, new information might emerge that would show some of these things do rate a classification as a carcinogen after all, so it pays to stay informed. But for now, although there are many probable or possible carcinogens out there, it is far more constructive to be aware of, and act upon, known and avoidable carcinogens like tobacco and viral infections for which there are vaccines, and to strive for a healthier lifestyle.

19. Which demographic groups have the highest risk of developing cancer?

Cancer incidence and mortality rates vary by country, geographic region, age, gender, race, socioeconomic status, and behavior patterns. According to the National Cancer Institute(NCI), the elderly are the demographic group with the highest risk of cancer. The median age of cancer diagnosis in the United States is sixty-six, and 60 percent of cancer patients are sixty-five or older. Whether it is the lifetime accumulation of exposure to things that could cause cancer, the declining effectiveness of the immune system, the increased chance of other chronic conditions, or simply the risk over time of cumulative random mutation, wear and tear simply adds up. Cancer is not an inevitable consequence of growing old, but it is most likely to happen as people get older.

Men as a demographic group also have increased risk, even adjusting for risk behaviors and exposure. Lifestyle is a big factor as men are more likely to engage in cancer-causing behaviors like tobacco or alcohol consumption, and they are more likely to be exposed to carcinogens while working in certain fields like construction and industrial settings.

But there are other, biological, theories as to why men are more prone to cancer than women. Studies have found a link between high levels of testosterone in the blood and certain cancers. And on a genetic level, women carry two copies of certain protective tumor suppressor genes because they have two X chromosomes, whereas men only have one, and are missing that extra line of defense. These chromosomal differences may explain why the disease sometimes develops differently in men and women and could give rise to more finely tuned treatment approaches. And finally, men are statistically less likely to seek medical care when they feel something is not right, which is not a surprise given how many of them refuse to ask for directions or read a manual.

The American Cancer Society's *Cancer Facts & Figures* is published annually and provides the most current information about cancer in the United States. It reported, in 2024, that overall rates of incidence and mortality have declined, but certain demographic groups are moving against these trends in a worrying way. These health disparities are defined as higher-than-average incidence and prevalence, earlier onset of disease, higher prevalence of risk factors and unhealthy behavior, and larger impact on daily functioning and quality of life, for a given population. These disparities are significant because, unlike age and gender, they are based on social factors that could be altered or improved.

The *Cancer Facts & Figures 2024* publication identified many disparities that stood out among demographic groups. Among racial and ethnic subgroups, African Americans men have the highest cancer death rate, a disparity largely driven by prostate cancer mortality. While African American women have a lower incidence of breast cancer than white women, they are more likely to die from it. African American, Hispanic/Latino, and American Indian/Alaska Native women have a higher incidence of cervical cancer than women in other ethnic groups. American Indian/Alaska Natives have the highest overall cancer incidence and mortality rates. These figures are influenced by exceptionally high rates of colorectal cancer among Alaska Native populations, which are among the highest in the world.

Geographically, three southern states have the highest cancer rates in the country, with Kentucky at the top of the list followed by Louisiana and Arkansas. People living in rural Appalachia have much higher rates of colorectal, lung, and cervical cancers than people living in urban areas in the same region. And although rural areas in general have lower incidence rates than urban areas, rural cancer death rates, especially for lung cancer, are higher. Regardless of race or ethnicity, people with less education are more likely to die prematurely from colorectal cancer. The American Cancer Society (ACS) report concluded that the lower the socioeconomic circumstances, the worse the cancer outcome. This is true not only in populations across the United States, but in countries all over the world.

Health inequities, which are defined as unjust and avoidable differences in health outcomes, are caused by a range of factors, social, environmental, and economic. The World Health Organization (WHO) calls these factors that impact health outcomes "social determinants of health." It defines these social determinants as "the conditions in which people are born, grow, work, live and age" as well as the policies, norms, and systems that shape those conditions.

It is no coincidence that the states with the highest incidence of cancer also have the highest proportion of people living below the poverty line. One of the main social determinants of poor health is poverty, which is associated with lack of safe housing, inadequate or no health insurance, and limited health literacy (because medical and insurance professionals tend to not communicate in simple clear language).

Poverty often goes hand in hand with a lack of access to quality medical care due to geographical barriers and lack of transportation. Economically depressed areas rarely have large medical centers, so lifesaving screening programs and therapeutic interventions are less accessible. These areas also tend to have a higher risk of environmental exposure to pollution or toxins depending on whether they are urban or industrial. Cancer risk is also higher in these places because there are higher rates of smoking and obesity.

Discrimination is another social determinant that is causing health disparities in the United States. American Indian/Alaska Natives are most likely to experience poverty, followed by African Americans. These groups also have the highest uninsured rates. Housing policies for minority groups have historically resulted in a lack of access to public transport, healthy foods, quality education, safe community spaces, and good medical care.

Minorities also experience a higher incidence of bias and discrimination from health care providers or systems. They tend to be underrepresented in clinical trials and biomedical research where participation rates are already very low, ranging from 3 to 16 percent. Having more diverse populations represented in clinical trials would help to improve health disparities but there are still many barriers to achieving this diversity. So ultimately, the care given to underrepresented groups may be less personalized to their needs.

Each edition of *Cancer Facts & Figures* includes a Special Section with an in-depth focus on timely cancer-related topics. The 2024 special section: *Cancer in people who identify as lesbian, gay, bisexual, transgender, queer or gender-non-conforming* revealed that people who identify as LGBTQ+ may be at increased risk of cancer because certain risk factors such as alcohol and tobacco use, obesity, and oncogenic viral infections like human papillomavirus

(HPV) and human immunodeficiency virus (HIV) are more common in that demographic group.

The report also stated that more than one in five LBGTQ+ individuals were likely to postpone or avoid medical attention based on negative past experience, or fear that the provider would refuse care. Discrimination and provider bias, as well as the fact that this demographic group is also statistically less likely to have health insurance, often lead to later diagnoses and poorer outcomes. Cancer statistics in this demographic group are generally focused only on increased risk because there is so little population-based data available about cancer rates by sexual orientation and gender identity.

Some demographic groups are culturally less likely to seek medical care, sometimes because of their practices and beliefs, and sometimes because of an inherent mistrust. Groups who are on the outskirts of society or who have been historically marginalized tend to have less trust in authorities, including medical authorities.

There can also be cultural or background barriers between a doctor and patient, where medical professionals are unaware of a potential dissonance between the way they speak to their patient and what the patient hears. Patients tend to be more comfortable and open about discussing their concerns with doctors to whom they can relate. And because health outcomes improve when doctors are fully informed, it is vital that patients and doctors learn how to better communicate with each other.

But cancer will not wait for sweeping social change, and health is of critical importance, both to the individual and to society. The statistics clearly underscore the fact that there are people at higher risk who are receiving less attention. The answers lie in addressing poverty, improving education, and increasing prevention awareness where and however it is appropriate. Meanwhile, individuals must keep advocating for their own health. They should get to know risks and ask questions, make healthy lifestyle choices, and access any and all preventive information and screenings their health care provides.

20. What organizations and public health initiatives exist, and how can they help prevent cancer?

Cancer prevention does not just save lives, it is critically important in easing the economic burden of cancer on the community and country. Public initiatives play an important role in preventing cancer and improving health outcomes by promoting awareness and education, offering vaccination, screening, and early detection programs, and helping people access preventive and supportive services and counseling. They also support research funding, and cancer registries. In the United States, several government and nongovernment organizations exist that are focused on cancer research, prevention, and early detection.

The National Cancer Institute (NCI) was established under the National Cancer Act of 1937. It is part of the National Institutes of Health and the government's primary agency for cancer research and training. The NCI is the largest funder of cancer research in the world. In 1971, President Nixon signed the National Cancer Act, declaring war on cancer, increasing the scope of research and funding of the NCI.

In 1973, the Surveillance, Epidemiology, and End Results (SEER) Program was established. Its goal was to collect and publish data from population-based registries in twenty-two different areas across the United States, and it collects information from about 800,000 cancer cases each year. The National Cancer Database (NCDB) was established in 1989, with the goal of tracking similar information directly from medical facilities.

The Centers for Disease Control and Prevention (CDC) established the National Program of Cancer Registries in 1992, which allowed them to provide funding and support across the country to start and improve local cancer registries and provide training and data processing systems to run them. One way for individuals to help these registries is with medical data and sample donation. Many people feel that if anything they can offer could potentially further cancer research, sharing their health data is worthwhile. All this data is critical for understanding, targeting, and addressing cancer-related issues.

The CDC also oversees the National Comprehensive Cancer Control Program which unites and supports cancer coalitions in every state, eight United States territories, and seven tribes and tribal organizations. They help these coalitions target cancers and risk factors that are specific to their communities, and promote prevention and screening. The goals of these programs are to educate the public about cancer prevention as well as increase screening rates and early diagnosis. The CDC also runs campaigns like Tips From Former Smokers which is aimed at addressing health disparities by helping people quit smoking regardless of who they are or where they live.

The Food and Drug Administration (FDA) is the government agency that now regulates the manufacture, distribution, and marketing of tobacco products, thanks to the 2009 Family Smoking Prevention and Tobacco Control Act. Their Center for Tobacco Products oversees the implementation of the Act by setting standards, reviewing premarket applications, and enforcing advertising restrictions.

The Environmental Protection Agency (EPA) protects public health and the environment by developing and enforcing safety regulations. Its focus is to prevent toxic exposure and reduce health risks. They established the National Primary Drinking Water Regulations to reduce exposure to carcinogens in water. SunWise is the EPA's health and environmental education program for sun safety with the goal of preventing skin cancer. The Occupational Safety and Health Administration (OSHA) has a similar mission to identify and combat workplace exposures by regulating carcinogens in industry and in the maritime and construction trades they regulate.

Some state-specific regulations exist to protect both the environment and consumers, such as Proposition 65 in California. Prop 65, which was passed in 1986, aims to prevent businesses from knowingly exposing people to substances that can cause cancer or birth defects. It requires clear warning labels on anything that contains these chemicals and also prohibits dumping them into drinking water or onto land where drinking water could be contaminated.

Many consumer products have been reformulated, public awareness has been raised about common carcinogens, and the government and industry have cooperated to create standards for many toxic chemicals. But critics cite the fact that businesses simply post meaningless warnings on their products instead of reformulating them in order to avoid the lawsuits that have multiplied as a result of Prop 65. New York and Washington have proposed or passed similar laws. Other states have raised the minimum age to purchase tobacco products to twenty-one, introduced legislation that prohibits minors from using ultraviolet tanning beds, and required health insurance policies to cover certain cancer screening tests.

The Persistent Poverty Initiative was launched in 2023 to address the structural and institutional factors of persistent poverty in the context of cancer. Coordinated by the NCI, the program hopes to create five new Centers for Cancer Control Research in Persistent Poverty Areas to improve intervention, prevention, follow-up care, and survivorship in their respective targeted low-income communities. Prevention will focus on reducing obesity and tobacco use, as well as improving nutrition, physical fitness, and living conditions. The research they conduct will inform future targeted campaigns and help train future investigators.

The two goals of the Cancer Moonshot, a White House cancer initiative, are to prevent more than 4 million cancer deaths by 2047, and to improve the experience of people who are affected by cancer. The Healthy People initiative is a plan released by the Department of Health and Human Services (HHS) every decade to improve the health of Americans. The goals set for 2030 by this initiative are to address heath disparities and reduce cancer risk through lifestyle changes and easy-to-access preventive care. Risk varies among different groups and understanding how and why these variances exist is the key to effective, targeted cancer prevention and intervention.

Many vaccination programs exist to ensure that everyone has access to the cancer preventing human papillomavirus (HPV) and hepatitis vaccines (HBV and HCV). These include the American Cancer Society's Mission: HPV Cancer Free initiative, and the CDC's Vaccines for Children program.

Many nongovernmental organizations like the American Cancer Society, the Prevent Cancer Foundation, the Livestrong Foundation, and the Susan G. Komen Foundation run advocacy and public awareness programs, community outreach programs, and raise money for cancer research. The American Cancer Society Cancer Action Network (ACS CAN) supports public policies to improve access to health coverage and prevent patients from incurring debt as a result of necessary cancer treatment.

World Cancer Day is held internationally every year on February 4 to raise awareness about cancer and encourage better prevention, detection, and treatment. Organizations like Union for International Cancer Control (UICC) and the World Health Organization (WHO) participate by mobilizing action to address the global cancer epidemic.

Consumer Reports is a nonprofit organization that focuses on product testing, investigative journalism, and public education. They have a policy of editorial independence and accept no advertising so they can offer unbiased reviews and warnings. They are consumer advocates who promote public health and are a good source for cancer prevention.

It is hard to quantify the effects of cancer prevention programs and initiatives. But, for example, the National Breast and Cervical Cancer Early Detection Program alone has funded programs that provided over 16 million breast and cervical cancer screening tests since 1991. These found nearly 78,000 breast cancers and more than 5,000 cervical cancers. Many of these are lives saved. Programs like this are good investments because prevention is always cheaper than intervention.

Diagnosing Cancer

21. What are the symptoms of cancer?

Cancer symptoms vary widely depending on the type, location, and stage of the disease. Some symptoms clearly point to the site of the developing cancer, while others can be vague and nonspecific. Some cancers cause no symptoms at all, particularly in early stages. Solid tumor cancer symptoms are different from blood cancer. Symptoms also depend on the individual's age and health.

The ways a disease manifests itself are known as symptoms and signs. Symptoms are the subjective feelings and perceptions of the patient; they cannot be detected or measured by a medical test. Pain, for example, is a symptom because only the patient can report on its location and severity. Signs, on the other hand, are objective indicators and can be directly observed and measured, like a fever or a lesion.

Symptoms and signs can occur as a direct result of cancer, such as swelling caused by a tumor. But often, they are an indirect or secondary effect, the body's reaction to what is happening to it. For example, a tumor may block airways leading to trapped secretions and cause an infection such as pneumonia, which is one of the indirect effects of lung cancer. Tumors can grow into, and press on, nearby tissues, organs, or nerves causing a variety of downstream symptoms. Most cancers cause many of the same general, nonspecific, symptoms and signs.

- Unexplained weight loss or gain: A loss or gain of 10 or more pounds, especially without trying, is a common sign of many cancers.
- Persistent fatigue: Exhaustion that does not improve with rest could be a symptom of anemia or low iron. It may be caused by gastrointestinal bleeding and is common with leukemia and colorectal cancers.
- Persistent fever: If a fever lasts a long time without any sign of infection or illness, or recurs often, it should be checked out. Some blood cancers can cause a fever that lasts for days or weeks, as well as heavy night sweats.

- Unexplained, chronic, and worsening pain: Bone cancer can cause pain early on. A tumor pressing on other tissues can cause pain that is difficult to pinpoint. Pain is a classic indication that something in the body is wrong.
- Visible skin changes: New growths, lumps, sores that do not heal (including sores in the mouth), changes in existing moles, and anything with an unusual shape, texture, or color, are all signs of various skin cancers. A lump in the scrotum can be a sign of testicular cancer. Skin darkening or yellowing, or areas of redness, itchiness, or increased hair growth anywhere on the body can indicate liver, ovarian, or kidney cancer.
- Unexplained or unusual bruising or bleeding: Tumors can make blood appear where it does not belong, like in the stool or urine. Nose bleeds can be a sign of nasal cavity or throat cancer but are also common with leukemia and lymphoma. Vaginal bleeding or discharge not associated with periods can be a sign of endometrial cancer.
- Swelling: Some cancers can cause swelling in the lymph nodes or thyroid. Breast cancer can cause lumps or thickening in the breast.
- Nagging cough or hoarseness: Lung cancer may cause persistent coughing, shortness of breath, and chest pain. Hoarseness can indicate a problem with the larynx or thyroid, and difficulty swallowing can be a sign of mouth or throat cancer.
- Bloating, indigestion, difficulty swallowing, and abdominal pain: Gastrointestinal cancers can cause lack of appetite and nausea, as well as changes in bowel habits like diarrhea and constipation. Ovarian cancer can cause pelvic or abdominal discomfort.
- Difficulty urinating: Prostate cancer is associated with difficulty urinating and lower back, hip, or thigh pain.
- Neurological symptoms: These can include seizures, vision, or hearing changes, and drooping of the face. Brain tumors can precipitate chronic headaches that do not respond to treatment.

While it is not necessary to remember all the possible signs and symptoms of cancer, it is wise to take notice of changes in or on the body that are new, that do not seem normal, or that do not go away. And if there are no symptoms but just a feeling something is wrong, it is still worth having a discussion with a medical professional who can advise on screenings or tests that might be appropriate. You know your body best and you should be your own strongest advocate when you need answers.

The vague nature of cancer symptoms makes it harder to find cancer when existing health conditions could be causing the same symptoms. This can result in cancer being diagnosed later. Even pregnancy can make symptoms of cancer appear to be related to general fatigue, hormone changes, or even hemorrhoids.

Often, these symptoms do end up indicating another health condition. But only a doctor and diagnostic testing can tell for sure. Symptoms for cancer may be generalized and vague, but if your symptoms have not improved after a week or two, they should absolutely not be ignored. Catching cancer at the earliest possible stage can save your life.

22. How is cancer found and diagnosed?

Cancer can be discovered in different ways. In the absence of symptoms, it can be found unintentionally, over the course of an unrelated examination, or during routine screening tests like a mammogram or a colonoscopy. When there are symptoms, like unexplained weight loss, fatigue, or bleeding, or physical changes like lumps, the patient will undergo a diagnostic workup.

After getting a rundown of symptoms and the patient's medical and family history, a medical provider will perform a physical examination to turn up any surface signs of the disease. Physical exams can consist of visual exams, during which doctors check for abnormal changes in skin color or texture, like lumps, lesions, and growths. Doctors will also palpate or press into the skin to feel for signs of disease like enlarged organs or lymph nodes. Physical exams include clinical breast exams and digital rectal exams.

No single test can accurately diagnose all cancers. Often many tests are needed to confirm or eliminate a cancer diagnosis. The most common diagnostic tests include laboratory tests, genetic tests, diagnostic imaging, endoscopic exams, and tumor biopsies.

Laboratory tests are run to show unusual changes in blood, urine, or other body fluids. Blood chemistry tests reveal how well various organs are functioning. A complete blood count (CBC) measures the number of white blood cells, red blood cells, and platelets, as well as the proportion and size of the red blood cells and the amount of hemoglobin they contain. Urinalysis and urine cytology measure the molecular contents of urine and look for abnormal cells that have been shed into the urinary tract. Sputum cytology does the same for mucus from the lung. Immunophenotyping is most often performed on blood or bone marrow to identify cancer cells based on certain markers. It can also monitor the progress of blood cancers like leukemia and lymphoma.

A test might look for tumor markers, which are any substances in the body, usually proteins, that could suggest the presence of cancer. They are found in blood, urine, stool, or tissues. Tumor markers are a by-product of, or a response to, a tumor. Certain genomic markers can also be used as tumor markers. Some might indicate a specific cancer, others are markers for multiple cancer types. Tumor markers are not completely accurate in that some individuals may have these markers in their blood for other reasons, and others may simply not produce detectable levels of them even if there is a tumor. The fluctuations of these levels over time may be more informative. They can be useful for diagnosis, staging, and deciding on treatment. They are also used to monitor the progress of treatment and whether a cancer has returned.

Liquid biopsies can be performed on blood samples to look for cancer cells or fragments of circulating tumor DNA that might have been released into the blood. They allow multiple samples to be taken over time with a simple noninvasive test and are mostly used to plan and monitor treatment. They can be used to detect cancer but are still not sensitive enough in many cases.

Increasingly, molecular and genetic testing is used to help clarify the nature of the cancer, distinguish between primary or secondary cancer, or identify a cancer of unknown primary origin. A cytogenic analysis, which looks for chromosomal changes, can be performed on samples of tissue, blood, bone marrow, or amniotic fluid. These changes might indicate certain cancers or genetic conditions.

A genetic test can check for inherited mutations in the patient. Tumor profiling, which sequences the DNA of biopsy samples to reveal mutations in the cancer itself, is becoming more common as more targeted therapies are developed. These tests can help indicate the aggressiveness of the cancer and what the prognosis is likely to be, as well as predict how it will respond to various treatments.

Inside the body, finding and diagnosing a tumor usually require imaging tests. These noninvasive tests are also used to stage cancer and monitor progress. Each imaging method provides a unique view of the body. The choice of test depends on tumor location, type, and the clinical questions being asked.

X-rays are a quick test that uses low level radiation to see all the internal structures of the body. They are mainly used to examine bones and joints. Different tissues will absorb different levels of radiation, making bones appear white and lungs appear dark.

Computed tomography (CT) scans use x-rays and a computer to create cross section images of the body. CT scans are more detailed than x-rays because the beam circles the body, creating images that can be viewed two-dimensionally or three-dimensionally. These scans expose patients to more radiation than regular x-rays but are administered less often.

Magnetic resonance imaging (MRI) produces detailed three-dimensional images using radio waves and strong magnetic fields. The machine consists of rings of magnets that form a tight tube around the patient. This produces a clear image but also causes some anxiety and claustrophobia.

Ultrasound imagery, or sonography, uses high-frequency sound waves reflected off structures within the body to create a real time image. A lymphangiogram is a kind of imaging that uses contrast dye and either x-rays or MRI to produce an image of the lymphatic system.

While CT and MRI scans show anatomy, positron emission tomography (PET) scans show cellular activity. PET scans use radioactively tagged glucose as a tracer that is injected into the body. When the tracer decays, it produces gamma rays that are detected by a scanner, which then produces a three-dimensional image. Because cancer cells are so hungry for glucose, the tracer lights up where it has become concentrated in a metabolically active tumor. This sign of abnormal cellular activity is how PET scans can differentiate between benign and malignant tumors. Bone scans work in a similar way, where a tracer is used to find evidence of bone destruction by tumor cells.

Once a tumor is detected, a biopsy is usually necessary to determine its nature. During a biopsy, a sample of the abnormal tissue is collected so it can be examined. Biopsies can be performed using a needle to draw out a sample. Fine needle aspiration biopsy is the removal of fluid or tiny fragments of tissue through a thin needle, whereas a core needle biopsy uses a long hollow needle to extract a narrow tube of tissue, called a core. Bone marrow biopsies are performed this way, aspirating a sample from the marrow or collecting a bone chip. Interventional radiology, like fluoroscopy, uses medical imaging, like x-ray or ultrasound to help precisely guide the process of needle aspiration. It is particularly necessary if the tumor is small and hard to reach.

Samples are also collected using various forms of endoscopy, a procedure in which a thin tube with a camera is inserted into the body to view internal organs. In a colonoscopy or sigmoidoscopy, the tube is inserted into the rectum. A colonoscopy examines the entire large intestine, while a sigmoidoscopy, which is less invasive, focuses on the lower part of the colon. In a cystoscopy, the tube goes through the urethra to examine the bladder. An esophagogastroduodenoscopy involves inserting the tube through the mouth to examine the esophagus, stomach, and upper part of the small intestine. In a bronchoscopy, the tube also goes through the mouth but continues into the lungs to inspect the airways. Another procedure, called endoscopic retrograde cholangiopancreatography, uses a similar approach but includes the insertion of a catheter into the bile ducts. Dye is then injected to make the liver, gallbladder, bile ducts, and pancreas visible on x-rays.

Tissue samples can also be collected surgically. Incisional biopsy is a procedure during which a portion of the tumor is removed for examination. Excisional biopsy is a procedure in which the entire tumor is removed, thereby saving the patient from possibly having to undergo a second procedure. A sentinel lymph node biopsy is the surgical removal of the lymph node closest to the tumor, into which the cancer is most likely to have spread.

There are various ways of removing samples of skin. A shave biopsy removes the very top layer of skin, whereas a punch biopsy involves taking a deeper core sample that includes the dermis and epidermis.

Biopsy samples are dissected and processed onto slides. They are then evaluated and examined under a microscope by a pathologist so they can identify the presence, type, and extent of the cancer. They examine the cells' location, appearance, and growth. Pathologists look for things like sheets of exceptionally large cells that are rapidly dividing, signs of tissue death, and signs of inflammation. Biopsies can reveal a specific diagnosis, what kind of cellular changes have taken place, what the tumor grade is, its severity or aggressiveness, and even suggest an appropriate course of treatment. At this point, cancer is confirmed. It can be staged, which establishes how far it has spread within the body, and graded, which is determined by the appearance and behavior of the cells. Often, nowadays, the sample will also undergo genomic testing to look for mutations and biomarkers.

23. How does cancer screening work?

Once a patient is diagnosed with cancer, what is known as the "clinical phase" of treatment begins. But prior to this milestone, during the "preclinical phase," the cancer has been developing from an initiating mutation to a varied cell population that is outcompeting normal cells. It is a process that can take one or two decades, sometimes longer. This phase gives us a huge opportunity to find and treat cancer early, by using cancer screening.

Cancer screenings are used to identify cancer or precancerous conditions in individuals who are apparently healthy and have no symptoms. This kind of proactive testing makes it possible to address cancer at the earliest possible stage, ideally before it has begun to spread. At this point, treatment is simpler, safer, and most effective.

Screening tests need to accomplish a few things to be considered worthwhile: they need to identify the disease before the onset of symptoms and offer more potential benefits than harm. Most importantly, effective cancer screening should result in lower mortality in screened individuals compared to unscreened individuals. Cancer screening tests are not considered diagnostic. Positive, abnormal, or suspicious test results mean follow-up diagnostic testing is required. Common recommended tests include breast, cervical, colorectal, and lung cancer screening.

The standard screening guidelines for most cancers recommend that people within specific age ranges get tested. Other candidates for screening include high-risk groups like people with a family history of cancer, with a known cancer related mutation, with weakened immune systems, or with certain lifestyle or environmental factors that would put them at higher risk. Different expert groups have different recommendations, but most agree that routine screenings should start between the ages of forty and fifty.

Cancer screenings vary based on the type of cancer they are targeting and can include physical exams, imaging, laboratory, and genetic tests. The most common screening test for breast cancer is mammography, an imaging test which shows the inside of the breast. It can detect small tumors and microcalcifications, tiny calcium deposits, which sometime indicate the presence of cancer. Film and digital mammography take an x-ray picture of the breast. Two-dimensional mammography uses x-rays to take pictures from two different angles. Digital breast tomosynthesis uses x-rays from many different angles to create a three-dimensional picture, which is the same principle as a CT scan but with less radiation. Many studies are still being conducted to determine what kind of breast cancer screening procedures (or combinations thereof) are the most effective.

During a mammogram, the breast is compressed between two plates and scanned. Compression reduces the chance of blurring and evens out the thickness of the breast tissue, which reduces the radiation dose. Mammograms are harder to interpret for women who have dense breast tissue, as both tissue and tumor appear similar in the scan. Breast density is not unusual, but it is a risk factor for breast cancer and people who perform mammograms are now required to tell women if they have dense breasts and how this impacts their test results. MRIs and ultrasound are also used to screen for breast cancer in women who have an elevated risk of developing the disease, or to further evaluate the results of a regular mammogram.

Cervical cancer is screened using a Pap test, also called Pap smear or cervical cytology. This test consists of using a small brush to collect a sample of cells from the cervix and examining them under the microscope to look for abnormalities. It is often used in conjunction with the human papillomavirus (HPV) test, which checks the cells for the DNA of certain strains of HPV that are associated with a high risk of cervical cancer.

Colorectal cancer can be screened using a variety of tests: a fecal occult blood test, colonoscopy, virtual colonoscopy, sigmoidoscopy, and a DNA stool test. The fecal occult blood test (FOBT) checks for signs of blood in the stool, which may be a sign of polyps or cancer.

Colonoscopy is the most common screening for colorectal cancer. During a colonoscopy, a flexible tube, containing a camera and a light, is inserted into the rectum and up into the colon. The tube also contains a small tool with which to remove polyps or tissue samples. These samples are then checked by a pathologist for signs of cancer.

A sigmoidoscopy uses a similar procedure to look into the sigmoid colon, it is quicker and less invasive than a colonoscopy but does not see as much. A virtual colonoscopy uses computed tomography (CT) scans to put together an image of the inside of the colon. A DNA stool test, like Cologuard, checks for cells with genetic changes that may be a sign of colorectal cancer. Although colonoscopy is the most effective and accurate way to screen for colorectal cancer, the less invasive tests might be more appropriate for people at average risk.

Lung cancer screening is recommended for people at high risk of developing the disease. It uses low-dose computed tomography (LDCT), which is a screening test that takes multiple x-ray images of the lungs and combines them using computers to create a comprehensive picture. Because there is less radiation exposure from LDCT scans, it is possible to use them more frequently as screening tests. The lower radiation means there is also lower resolution, or less image clarity, but it is effective enough to identify nodules and tumors in low-density tissue like lungs.

The prostate-specific antigen (PSA) test is a simple blood test used to screen for prostate cancer. PSA is a tumor marker, a protein which is produced by the prostate gland. High PSA levels are also associated with other benign conditions such as enlarged prostate and prostatitis. If testing shows high levels of PSA as well as prostate enlargement, the next step is usually watchful waiting and taking more PSA measurements over time, because prostate cancer is often very slow growing. The PSA test is not definitive, its rate of false positives is around 75 percent. The test itself is simple and relatively safe, and it is a convenient monitoring tool. The risks associated with it are related to the diagnostic tests that follow a positive test result, including prostate biopsy, overdiagnosis, and overtreatment, as well as treatment complications such as incontinence and erectile dysfunction.

Genetic or molecular testing is not diagnostic, nor is it really cancer screening, but it is considered a risk assessment tool that can guide more frequent or more targeted screening. These are blood or saliva tests given to people with a strong family history or known genetic predisposition for mutations like BRCA1 and BRCA2 or Lynch syndrome.

Other screening tests for cancer exist, but they are not currently recommended by organizations that create screening guidelines because they are less reliable, are still being studied, or have simply not proven to lower overall mortality. They are sometimes offered, however, especially to people who are at higher risk of a particular cancer.

For example, there is no reliable screening test for ovarian cancer in women who do not have symptoms. But there are tests used to monitor treatment or recurrence that can also be used for women who have the BRCA2 mutation or other elevated risk factor. These tests are the CA-125, which measures the levels of a tumor marker called cancer antigen 125 in the blood, and an imaging test called a transvaginal ultrasound.

Current research is focusing on refining screening based on individual risk factors rather than just age. Being able to narrow the parameters for each individual would improve early detection rates while reducing unnecessary procedures in low-risk groups. This approach also gives medical professionals the opportunity to assess their patients' lifestyle and environmental risk factors like diet or obesity. This focus on intervention could have a huge impact on cancer outcomes.

Multi-cancer early detection (MCED) tests, like Galleri or CancerSEEK, are liquid biopsies that are meant to detect multiple cancers through a simple blood sample. They measure biomarkers like circulating tumor cells, tumor DNA, mutations, and proteins. Studies show that many MCEDs have great potential and are unlikely to produce false positives. But while they show promise, their sensitivity varies by test and cancer type. They are better at detecting late-stage cancers than early-stage, which is less beneficial.

Although they are minimally invasive tests, they are not always superior. The Shield blood test for colon cancer, which was recently approved by the Food and Drug Administration (FDA), identifies only about 13 percent of polyps. A colonoscopy identifies 95 percent. Additionally, these tests are rarely covered by insurance and can be very expensive. Finally, it is still unknown if they will reduce overall cancer mortality, which is ultimately the goal of cancer screening. There is not sufficient evidence at this time that they will replace standard cancer screenings, even though Congress is looking at legislation that would allow Medicare coverage for MCED tests, once the FDA approves them. As the technology develops, there is little doubt they will improve in sensitivity and accuracy.

Another emerging technology in cancer screening is the use of artificial intelligence (AI) to identify cancer in medical imaging from mammograms to MRIs. Because AI is capable of analyzing an image based on the available data from thousands of images on which it is trained, results are both faster and more precise. The FDA has already approved AI-assisted tools to help detect brain, breast, lung, prostate, skin, and thyroid cancer.

There are many methods of screening, but only a few of them are recommended by regulatory agencies like the United States Preventive Services Task Force (USPSTF) and other organizations like the American Cancer Society (ACS). This is because, ultimately, for cancer screening tests to reduce mortality, they must reliably find the cancer, and there must be an effective treatment to address it.

Cancer screening offers the benefit of possible early detection and intervention, and an improved prognosis. It can detect cancer early, increasing the likelihood of successful treatment. In some cases, it can even prevent cancer by identifying and removing precancerous lesions. It also offers psychological benefits, like peace of mind. And finally, there is a huge cost savings to catching cancer early because late-stage cancer is the most expensive stage to treat.

However, not all screening tests have the same degree of accuracy, and most have some degree of risk. False positives, which wrongly suggest the presence of cancer, can lead to stress and unnecessary procedures. While false negatives, test results that miss the presence of cancer, may delay diagnosis. Radiation exposure and invasive follow-up tests add further risk, and overdiagnosis of slow-growing cancers can result in overtreatment. Addressing cancers in these cases might not provide a clear survival benefit since they might never have become life-threatening in the first place. It might also mean going through treatment and side effects which might not even have been necessary.

And early detection is useless if there is no way to diagnose or treat the disease. In the case of rare and aggressive cancers, early detection will probably not improve the outcome anyway, and the patient has received a distressing diagnosis about which they can do nothing. Sometimes screening is more informational than actionable.

It is important to understand your own personal risk factors and weigh risks and benefits when it comes to cancer screening. People who have no symptoms and are at average risk should follow recommended screening guidelines. A medical professional can use risk assessment tools to find out who might be at higher risk and adjust the screening schedule as needed.

24. How is cancer staged?

Cancer staging is the process of identifying how much cancer is present and how far it has spread within the body. Staging gives a comprehensive picture of the disease which is used to determine possible treatment strategies and help predict survival rates. Staging is also a standardized and consistent way to describe cancer and is useful for comparing conditions among different patient populations. It is the most powerful predictor of outcome for a cancer patient.

A cancer is typically staged at the time of diagnosis and this initial clinical staging is the one that is considered when projecting survival rates. Sometimes, it is staged again after further examination or treatment. If the tumor is removed surgically, additional details may be revealed. This type of examination is called pathological staging.

Staging might also be done after treatment to assess the cancer's response, or if the cancer returns or progresses. The new stage classification will be added to the original stage, but it will not replace it. Stage is determined using things like physical examination, imaging tests, endoscopy, biopsy, and blood tests. Other factors that are considered in cancer staging include the patient's age, the tumor's location, grade, cell type, and levels of tumor markers or biomarkers in the blood.

There are different methods of staging cancer, but the most common is the TNM system. This standardized system, which stands for Tumor, Node, and Metastasis, is maintained and updated by the American Joint Committee on Cancer, and the Union for International Cancer Control. This kind of staging applies mainly to carcinomas, which account for 80 to 90 percent of all cancers. The TNM system assigns a letter or number to describe three basic elements. T describes the extent of the primary tumor, N describes the status of the lymph nodes located near the primary tumor, and M describes the presence or absence of metastasis in distant parts of the body. Each category can be assigned a letter or number, notations which may vary slightly when describing different cancers.

For tumors, "TX" indicates there is no information about the tumor, or it cannot be measured. "T0" indicates no tumor is present. "Tis" means the cancer is in situ, or a pre-cancer, and has not penetrated into deeper layers of tissue. Numbers after the T (T1 to T4) describe the tumor's size or the extent of its spread. The higher the T number, the more the tumor has developed.

For lymph nodes, "NX" means there is no information about the nodes, or they cannot be assessed. "N0" indicates no spread to the nearby lymph nodes. Numbers after the N (N1 to N3) indicate the extent that the lymph nodes have been affected by the cancer. The higher the N number, the more the lymph nodes have been affected.

For metastasis, "MX" means metastasis cannot be assessed. "M0" means there is no distant metastasis. "M1" means the cancer has spread to distant tissues in the body.

So, for example, a small tumor that has spread to the lymph nodes but nowhere else in the body, might be described as "T2 N1 M0." Lower case letters are sometimes used to refine the number categories, so a lung cancer described as "M1a" has spread to the other lung, "M1b" indicates it has spread to another part of the body, and "M1c" means it has spread to several areas of the body. Other notations might include whether the staging is clinical or pathological, and whether it was done after therapy, or after recurrence or progression.

Number staging systems use the TNM values and other factors to divide cancers into four stages. These stages, numbered 1 through 4, are usually written out in Roman numerals.

Stage I: The cancer is relatively small and contained where it first appeared.

Stage II: The cancer is larger but still localized. With certain cancers, stage II indicates some spread into nearby lymph nodes.

Stage III: The cancer is regional, larger than in stage II and it may be spreading into surrounding tissues. Cancer cells can be present in the nearby lymph nodes.

Stage IV: The cancer has spread from its point of origin to another organ or distant area of the body. This is metastatic or secondary cancer.

These categories are sometimes further divided into A, B, C, or D to describe the aggressiveness of the disease. So, for example, a stage IIIA cancer is less aggressive than a stage IIIB cancer.

Stage 0 is sometimes used to describe a carcinoma in situ, which is a precancerous change or noninvasive cancer. This group of abnormal cells too small to be a tumor could develop into cancer in the future. There is a stage V classification, but it is rarely used except to describe some rare tumors.

Some cancers are staged using other systems, such as the Ann Arbor staging system which is used to describe lymphomas. The International Federation of Gynecologists and Obstetricians have their own staging system for female reproductive cancers that is similar to TNM staging. Brain cancers do not have formal staging because they do not normally spread. Leukemias have already spread throughout the body through the circulatory system but are sometimes staged based on white blood cell levels, the condition of the lymph nodes, and the condition of the liver and spleen.

The National Cancer Institute's Surveillance, Epidemiology and End Results (SEER) Summary Staging system is a simplified version of cancer staging used for statistical purposes such as tracking survival rates. It is straightforward and is not updated or changed over time, which allows trends to be followed for many years. The basic SEER Summary Stages are roughly the same as the numeric staging system. Cancers are classified as in situ, localized, regional, distant, and unknown.

Staging does have some drawbacks, because a cancer diagnosis can be far more nuanced and ambiguous than the classification models would suggest. It is based on population studies which is why it is particularly useful for research but does not always reflect the individual. It can also be somewhat arbitrary. Its value is in providing a general framework which is then enhanced by the information gathered in clinical testing, pathology, imaging, and increasingly, with molecular profiling.

25. How is cancer graded?

Whereas a tumor's stage refers to size and spread, tumor grade refers to the appearance of the tumor's cells under the microscope. Grading assesses how the tumor is likely to behave based on how normal or abnormal the cells look. It is also an important tool for predicting how a tumor will respond to various treatment approaches. This kind of grading applies mainly to carcinomas, which account for 80 to 90 percent of all cancers. Tumor grade is a predictor of patient outcome, as low-grade tumors have a better prognosis than high-grade tumors.

To establish grade, a sample of the tumor's tissue is collected with a biopsy and examined under the microscope. A pathologist will evaluate the level of differentiation in the cells, as well as their architecture and organization.

Differentiation refers to how cells gradually become specialized and perform different functions. As cancer progresses, the cells divide faster and more uncontrollably. They are incapable of specializing and start looking very distinct from the normal tissue around them. The degree of differentiation can vary within a tumor, so grade is based on the most poorly differentiated cells. Lower-grade cancers show more differentiation and still resemble their tissue of origin, whereas higher-grade cancers have less differentiation. Most solid tumors are assessed for grade using a four-tiered scale.

Grade 1: The cells in a grade 1 tumor are still well differentiated and slow growing. They still look like the healthy cells that surround them. Grade 1 is a low-grade tumor.

Grade 2: The cells in a grade 2 tumor are moderately differentiated. They look slightly abnormal. This is an intermediate grade.

Grade 3: The cells in a grade 3 tumor are poorly differentiated and lack architecture and structure. This is a high-grade tumor.

Grade 4: The cells in a grade 4 tumor are undifferentiated. They are so primitive looking they are referred to as anaplastic, or without form. These tumors grow aggressively and spread fast. Grade 4 is a high-grade tumor.

The term "grade X" is applied when a tumor is insufficiently tested, or the test results were unclear or inconclusive. This grade is undetermined.

Some cancers use their own specialized grading systems. Prostate cancer is graded using the Gleason score, which rates the cells on a scale of 2 to 10 with 10 being the highest grade. The score is obtained by combining the grades of the two most common cell patterns in the tumor.

Breast cancer is graded using different scoring systems like the Nottingham Histologic score and the Bloom-Richardson score. These systems look at three factors, the amount of gland formation, the nuclear features of the cells, and the mitotic activity, or rate of cell division. Grades are assigned to each factor and added up to grade the overall tumor.

Kidney cancers are graded using the Fuhrman grading system, a four-tier system which assesses the cells based on size, shape, and DNA structure.

Certain blood cancers have their own grading systems as well. Non-Hodgkin lymphomas are graded as low, intermediate, or high, depending on their rate of growth.

Tumor grading is a subjective evaluation, the degree of differentiation in a tumor's cells is an arbitrary point on a continuum. This gives rise to some differences and discrepancies between pathologists' findings. Artificial intelligence (AI) and deep learning models show a lot of promise in enhancing the accuracy and consistency of cancer grading, especially in cases of breast, prostate, lung, colorectal, and brain cancer. But at time of publication, it is still mostly used in research and for diagnostic support.

26. Why is it important to find cancer early?

Detecting cancer early is a critical factor in improving survival rates. Studies and systematic reviews have found that many cancers, including colorectal, breast, lung, and cervical, have a better prognosis the earlier they are found. Finding cancer early can save lives.

Successful early detection relies on screening and early diagnosis. Screening is a means of finding cancer in a symptomless population using tests like colonoscopies and mammograms. Early diagnosis is focused on correctly identifying disease in symptomatic patients as early as possible. And with genetic testing, high-risk groups can be identified and proactively monitored.

Early detection often results in increased survival rates because it provides the best chance of successful preventive intervention. Late-stage cancers have much lower survival rates. According to the National Cancer Institute's Surveillance, Epidemiology and End Results (SEER) database, an early stage localized non squamous cell lung cancer's five-year survival rate is 65 percent. The five-year survival rate for the same cancer at a late or distant stage is 9 percent. In addition, early-stage cancers can be addressed with much less aggressive or invasive treatment, which means shorter recovery times. It also means fewer or less intense side effects, and better quality of life. (See Question 27—What is the prognosis for someone diagnosed with cancer?)

Treating late-stage cancer is also substantially more expensive than addressing it at an early stage. A 2018 systematic review examining the global treatment costs of breast cancer by stage found that the cost of stage IV breast cancer treatment was 109 percent higher than stage I. This increase is usually driven by the cost of more intensive and more frequent therapies.

A 2023 research paper published in the *Journal of the American College of Surgeons* underscored the critical nature of early detection. They found that an unintended consequence of the Covid-19 pandemic was how much it disrupted routine cancer care. The research showed a significant drop in cancer incidence rates in 2020 compared to pre-pandemic rates, which does not mean fewer people got cancer, it means fewer people were diagnosed. This suggests many people may currently be harboring undiagnosed disease as a result. The pandemic had a profound impact on early detection because hospitals were overwhelmed, and non-emergency procedures and screenings were postponed. Referral rates fell sharply, resulting in subsequent delays in timely diagnosis and treatment. The full effects of this disruption in screening schedules may take years to become apparent, with greater than anticipated numbers of late-stage cancer diagnoses.

But early detection is only effective when patients are actually getting screened and diagnosed. The target participation rates for cancer screening are not being met in the United States. The Centers for Disease Control and Prevention (CDC) published a paper in 2023 which revealed that one in four adults were not up to date with breast, cervical, and colorectal cancer screening recommendations. Screening rates fall short for a number of reasons such as access to health care, socioeconomic factors, and lack of awareness.

Early detection is an advantage when dealing with the most common and commonly screened cancers like breast, lung, colorectal, and cervical, because the tests are generally reliable, and the treatments are generally beneficial. But early detection is useless if there is no way to diagnose or treat the disease, and sometimes screening is more informational than actionable. If early detection identifies an indolent, or slow-growing, cancer, there is a risk of overdiagnosis and overtreatment. Addressing this kind of cancer might not provide a clear survival benefit since it might never have become life-threatening in the first place. And in the case of rare and aggressive cancers, early detection might not improve the outcome anyway. Screening recommendations factor in these potential benefits and risks, which is why rare and fatal cancers are not routinely screened. Screening for cancers like pancreatic or liver cancer is only done for people who have a known risk.

Education and public awareness should encourage people to be proactive about finding cancer early. Because it can lead to a timelier diagnosis and earlier treatment, early detection saves lives and reduces suffering. It also cuts treatment costs and relieves the patient and the health care system of the heavier burden presented by late-stage disease.

27. What is the prognosis for someone diagnosed with cancer?

Prognosis is the likely course of the disease, or the outlook for the patient once they have a diagnosis. The prognosis for someone diagnosed with cancer is highly individual and depends on several factors, such as the type of cancer, the stage at diagnosis, the treatment options, and the age and overall health of the patient.

Prognosis is often expressed as a five-year survival rate. Cancer statistics use a five-year survival rate as a percentage to describe how many people are likely to survive the disease for at least five years after diagnosis. If a certain type of cancer at a certain stage has a survival rate of 70 percent, it means 70 out of 100 people who have that cancer at that particular stage are expected to be alive after five years. The five-year survival rate is a statistical overview and does not take into account the patient's age or health, how they might respond to treatment or whether the cancer might come back. These numbers are only based on the stage of the cancer at diagnosis. If the cancer is subsequently restaged, the statistics no longer apply.

A cancer-specific survival rate is the percentage of people who are alive five years after a specific cancer diagnosis. It is measured by counting only the deaths that were directly attributed to that specific diagnosis and does not include patients who died from other causes. This is also called "net cancer survival."

Disease-free survival is the percentage of patients who have no signs of cancer for a certain period of time after treatment. It is also called "recurrence-free" or "progression-free" survival. The relative cancer survival rate compares people with a certain cancer diagnosis to people of the same sex, age, and race, who do not have that diagnosis. This shows how much a specific cancer shortens lifespan.

These survival rates are a useful tool for researchers and clinicians. And although cancer survival rates do not predict your personal life expectancy, they are an estimate of what could happen and when. Some patients want to know their odds. They want to make plans so they want to know how long they might have. But some patients do not react well to being told how long they are likely to survive and prefer not to feel the pressure of what is essentially a statistical guess. If an average survival time is twelve months, for example, it means that half of all patients with this diagnosis lived less than twelve months and half lived more than twelve months, it does not mean this is how much time the patient has to live.

The stage at diagnosis is probably the most critical factor in assessing a prognosis. Earlier stage cancers typically have better outcomes than later stages, which is why early detection is so vital in many cases. The grade of the tumor, or the appearance of its cells, is also related to prognosis, with higher-grade tumors being associated with poorer survival rates. Late stage and high grade are associated with metastasis, which makes any kind of treatment less likely to be effective.

Age is another key factor in determining a cancer prognosis. Younger and healthier individuals tend to have a better prognosis because they can better tolerate aggressive treatments and harsh side effects. An older patient is also more likely to have a longer history of exposure and a weaker immune system. Recent research suggests that age-related changes occur in the tumor microenvironment which may reduce the effectiveness of the treatments.

Older patients also tend to have comorbidities—two or more medical conditions that are present simultaneously. A 2024 article published in the *Journal of the National Cancer Institute* revealed that more than 90 percent of older adults with cancer have one or more comorbidities, such as high blood pressure, cardiovascular disease, obesity, and diabetes. Having these chronic conditions while undergoing cancer treatment is much harder on the system and makes managing the disease more complex. Overall health is a critical determinant in how well a cancer patient will cope.

Different cancers have vastly different survival rates. Some skin cancers, like basal cell carcinomas, have a 100 percent five-year survival rate when detected and treated early. So, the prognosis depends on whether the cancer is slow growing or aggressive, whether it tends to be localized or metastasized. Prognosis is also affected by the cancer's risk of coming back, or recurrence. Triple-negative breast cancer, for example, has a higher recurrence rate than other types of breast cancer, so this diagnosis generally has a worse prognosis.

Treatment options affect prognosis because some cancers are simply more difficult to treat than others. Cancers that are advanced or aggressive may be considered untreatable, such as glioblastoma, a form of brain cancer that is resistant to most treatments and for which complete surgical removal is rarely an option. Other cancers, like thyroid cancer, have many treatment options and can usually be treated successfully.

With the advances in precision medicine, an approach to treatment that considers genetic or molecular profiling to provide more personalized interventions, patients have the benefit of receiving more effective treatment and fewer side effects. While standardized classifications like stage and grade provide a general framework for treatment and prognosis, this molecular data allows vulnerabilities in the cancer itself to be identified and targeted. It can also predict how a tumor is likely to respond to, or resist, certain therapies. But many cancer therapies still have significant side effects and the individual's response to a cancer treatment and how well they can tolerate it are also significant factors.

28. What are the screening guidelines in the United States?

Cancer screening makes it possible to address the disease at the earliest possible stage because this is when treatment is simpler, safer, and most effective. In the United States, cancer screening guidelines are developed by several organizations, including the United States Preventive Services Task Force (USPSTF), the American Cancer Society (ACS), and the National Comprehensive Cancer Network (NCCN). These organizations' guidelines do not always agree, but they all base their recommendations on reviews of scientific literature, public health considerations, expert consensus, and a careful weighing of the benefits versus the harms of screening. The main recommended screenings are for breast, cervical, and colorectal cancer. Additionally, prostate and lung cancer screenings are recommended for individuals with an elevated risk.

For a screening test to be recommended, it needs to be able to identify the disease before the onset of symptoms and offer more potential benefits than harm. The risks are the same as for any procedure or testing: stress, injury, and exposure. Screening can also lead to further tests which may be increasingly risky or invasive. Most importantly, effective cancer screening should result in lower mortality in screened individuals compared to unscreened individuals.

Breast cancer screening—The ACS screening guidelines for breast cancer are that women between the ages of forty and forty-four may start getting a mammogram every year if they choose. Women forty-five to fifty-four should get a mammogram every year. Women fifty-five and older can continue with their annual mammograms or switch to every other year. Screening should continue as long as the woman is healthy and expected to live at least ten more years.

For women at higher risk of breast cancer, the ACS recommends getting a breast MRI and a mammogram every year, typically starting at age thirty. This includes women who have a family history of breast cancer, a known high-risk genetic mutation, like BRCA1 or BRCA2, certain genetic syndromes, or women who have had chest radiation therapy before the age thirty.

The USPSTF recommends mammography screening for women aged forty to seventy-four years every two years, as they have concluded that screening every two years has a more favorable balance of benefits to harms. They also recommend that clinicians use risk assessment tools on women with a personal or family history of breast, ovarian, tubal, or peritoneal cancer to determine if genetic testing would be appropriate.

Cervical cancer screening—The ACS recommends cervical cancer screening for women aged twenty-five to sixty-five. They should have a primary human papillomavirus (HPV) test every five years, screening with a co-test that combines an HPV test with a Pap test every five years, or a Pap test alone every three years. After age sixty-five, the recommendation is to keep testing only if there have been previous abnormal results, or any treatment for cervical cancer or pre-cancer.

The USPSTF recommends women aged twenty-one to twenty-nine be tested every three years with a Pap test alone. Women aged thirty to sixty-five years should be tested every three years with a Pap test and every five years with an HPV test, or every five years with the co-test.

Colorectal cancer screening—The ACS and USPSTF recommend that people at average risk of colorectal cancer start regular screenings at age forty-five, a recent change made due to a sharp rise in early-onset colorectal cancer incidence. The recommendation is to use stool-based tests every one to three years, colonoscopy every ten years, or virtual colonoscopy or sigmoidoscopy every five years. Abnormal results from any non-colonoscopy test should be followed up with a colonoscopy. Screening should continue through age seventy-five, at which point the decision to screen should be based on preference, history, life expectancy, and overall health.

The ACS does not have specific recommendations for people at elevated risk of colorectal cancer beyond getting earlier and more frequent testing. People at high risk include those with a personal or family history of colorectal cancer or polyps, a personal history of bowel disease, a known family history of a hereditary syndrome like Lynch syndrome, or a personal history of radiation to the abdomen or pelvis due to a prior cancer.

Lung cancer screening—Both the USPSTF and ACS recommend low-dose computed tomography (LDCT) for the early detection of lung cancer in high-risk individuals. Specifically, people between the ages of fifty and eighty who have a twenty or higher pack-year history of smoking, who smoke currently, or who quit within the last fifteen years. A pack-year is calculated by multiplying the number of packs per day by the number of years smoked. So, a twenty pack-year history means they smoked a pack per day for twenty years, or two packs per day for ten years, or a half pack per day for forty years.

Prostate cancer screening—The USPSTF selectively recommends prostate cancer screening for men aged fifty-five to sixty-nine years using the PSA test. The recommendation is selective, meaning it is up to the doctor and patient to decide, because although the screening offers a small potential benefit for some men, more men experience the potential harms.

The ACS recommends that men aged fifty and older, of average risk, should have a conversation with their provider before making an informed decision.

People at a higher risk, including African American men, men with an inherited mutation, or a family history of prostate cancer, should have this conversation starting ages forty to forty-five.

The National Comprehensive Cancer Network (NCCN) recommends starting the conversation with your doctor about screening at age fifty for average risk and repeating the test every one to four years depending on the PSA level. For men at a higher risk, they recommend annual screening starting age forty.

The decision to have prostate cancer screening is generally left up to the doctor and patient because, although the tests can detect more prostate cancers, they do not seem to affect overall mortality. Prostate cancer is generally very slow growing and often needs no immediate intervention. And while PSA tests are simple blood tests, they can lead to overtreatment and potential complications like incontinence and erectile dysfunction from biopsies or surgery. Prostate cancer is diagnosed in only about 25 percent of people who have had a biopsy following a positive PSA test, and false positives are common. Some alternatives to the traditional PSA test are being investigated, such as looking at PSA density or PSA doubling time. Other prostate cancer antigens, such as urinary biomarkers, are also currently being studied.

People who identify as a gender different from the one they were born with should have a frank discussion with a medical professional about which kinds of screening would be appropriate.

Cancer screening tests are constantly being studied in clinical trials to assess their safety and efficacy. These studies are the basis for screening recommendations because the tests need to be more than simply effective. Ideally, screening should provide a lead time, a way to improve chances of survival. But in reality, some cancers are so aggressive that even an early diagnosis may already be too late, and other cancers are so slow growing that screening makes no difference because the cancer would never affect the patient anyway.

The World Health Organization (WHO) recommends that screening programs should only be implemented when their effectiveness is clear, when resources are sufficient, when facilities exist to confirm the diagnosis and ensure proper treatment, and when the prevalence of the disease is high enough to justify the cost of screening.

Organizations that make screening recommendations assess populations for their cancer risk, set age ranges, and determine frequency of testing. They want to optimize early detection without risking overdiagnosis. This is why screening tests for some other cancers, like endometrial biopsies, only apply to high-risk populations. They review scientific literature and update the recommendations as needed. When developing screening guidelines, they must also factor in the resources available to support administering the test and reaching target screening participation rates.

The USPSTF grades various screening methods based on data related to the effectiveness of screening, and the strength of the evidence of benefit versus harm. The grades are A—Recommended, B—Recommended, with moderate net benefit, C—Selectively Recommended, D—Not Recommended, or I—Uncertain. They routinely update the recommendations to reflect new evidence.

A cancer screening test should, above all, decrease mortality from that cancer. It should be sensitive, meaning it can correctly identify individuals *with* the cancer. It should also be specific, in that it should be able to correctly identify individuals *without* that cancer. This is to minimize the chances of false positives and false negatives, which is where many of the potential harms of screening arise.

Whether or not the test is effective depends on its predictive value, as well as how common that cancer is in a given population. In a low-risk population, the chance of finding cancer is much lower, in which case the risk of screening and possible follow-up testing, including radiation exposure and invasive biopsies, outweighs the possible benefit. And finally, testing a low-risk population is a burden on the health care system that offers very little return. Ultimately, screening recommendations are in place to provide the greatest health benefits to the greatest number of people.

Treating Cancer

29. Can cancer be cured?

Because cancer is an umbrella term for hundreds of diseases that are genetically distinct, there is no "cure" for cancer. From a patient's point of view, a cure (or treatment) for cancer often means there is a mechanism for long-term survival after diagnosis. Curing cancer depends on the type of cancer, its stage and location, treatment options and their effectiveness, how the cancer responds to therapy, and the patients' overall health and age.

The term "cure" is difficult to pin down in the field of oncology because it implies the cancer is permanently eradicated and there is long-term survival without recurrence. Recurrence means the cancer has come back. A patient can be considered cured of cancer if their life expectancy once again aligns with the general population's.

But the term "cure" is rarely used because it is often impossible to tell if any cancer cells are still in the body. This is why doctors will more often use the term "remission." Remission is the time during which the cancer is under control or responding to treatment. Partial remission indicates the cancer is responding to treatment but is not completely gone. Complete remission means the signs and symptoms of the cancer are gone, and tests are revealing no presence of cancer cells. If the patient is in complete remission for five years or more, some doctors might use the word "cured," because the longer the patient remains cancer free, the less likely it will return. It is possible that there can be dormant cancer cells somewhere in the body, but when cancer comes back, it generally does so within the first five years after treatment.

Cancer is more likely to be cured if it is caught early, when it is still stage I or stage II cancer. A complete surgical removal followed by treatment, if necessary, can often lead to complete remission. Certain types of cancer are also more responsive to treatment, such as testicular and thyroid. With current treatments, even advanced Hodgkin lymphoma has high cure rates. But even with remission, some cancers can return, sometimes years later. Cancers like triple-negative breast cancer have high recurrence rates and are harder to treat long-term.

When cancer is not changing it is called stable disease. When it grows or spreads it is called cancer progression. Progression is usually a sign that not all the cancer was eliminated, or that it developed a resistance to the treatment. This is also true for cancers that have reappeared or recurred.

Advanced-stage cancers like stage IV lung or pancreatic cancer, and aggressive cancers like malignant mesothelioma or glioblastoma, are generally considered incurable. But some of them are still treatable. Rather than focusing on a cure, treatment is centered around prolonging survival by managing the disease as much as possible. At this point, treatment can still shrink a tumor, slow its development, and relieve symptoms. In some cases, cancer is treated long-term with ongoing monitoring and follow-up care. Remission and survival rates, on the whole, show that people are not only living longer in remission, but also living longer with their cancer, which is being treated as a chronic condition.

Cure can also depend on the location of the cancer. Some areas of the body are easy and relatively safe to access surgically. Small tumors on the skin, breast, or testicles, for example, can be completely removed. But some places in the body present too high a risk for surgical removal. Tumors near blood vessels, or certain parts of the brain, or tumors that are thread-like rather than a solid mass, are often considered inoperable. In this case, other treatments like radiation, chemotherapy, or immunotherapy are recommended.

Tumors are hard to address if they cannot be removed, and they present several challenges to these therapies. They often have chaotic blood vessel structures and high internal pressure, which make it hard for drugs to penetrate. Cancer cells can secrete molecules on their surface that are capable of switching off the immune response, effectively making them invisible to the immune system. They adapt and evolve faster than the healthy cells around them. And so, treatments can fail, or stop working over time, because cancer cells evolve and adapt in unpredictable ways.

Two individuals with the same cancer may not respond to the same therapy in the same way. Even in the same tumor, the cells are not all identical and may have different mutations. One of the reasons cancers stop responding to treatment is tumor heterogeneity. This refers to the different subpopulations of cancer cells that exist within a tumor. Each subpopulation has different genetic characteristics and growth patterns. And most importantly, each subpopulation might respond to treatment differently, with non-responsive cells surviving and multiplying, which is how the disease can become treatment resistant.

Most cancer therapies are notoriously hard on the system, and research is constantly trying to balance their effectiveness with their toxicity. Ultimately, cancer cells are still human cells, and although the programming may be corrupted, they still have the same programming, so to speak. So, as effective as a cancer treatment is against cancer cells, it is going to be just as devastating to healthy cells. Although not all advanced cancers respond to therapy, all patients experience some toxic side effects.

This is why age and overall health are critical factors in the likelihood of a patient being cured. Physical resilience is required in the face of side effects like cardiovascular issues, blood clots, impaired organ function, or nerve damage. Younger patients are also less likely to have comorbidities, or preexisting conditions, which can make it harder to tolerate certain treatments. People with a strong immune system will be better equipped to fight infections, not to mention recovering from surgery faster and with fewer complications. Undergoing multiple therapies requires stamina, and patients who are frail or weak are less likely to complete their treatments.

If cancer reaches a stage when it cannot be cured or controlled with any treatment, it is considered terminal. The disease is leading to death, and the main goal is palliative care. Palliative care is not meant to treat the disease, it is meant to alleviate symptoms, provide comfort, and preserve quality of life as much as possible.

So, are we getting better at treating cancer? In 2022, there were more than 18 million cancer survivors living in the United States. The National Institutes of Health (NIH) projects that by 2040, there will be 26 million. This reflects an increase in population, aging population in particular, but also demonstrates the slow but steady ways we are improving how we fight and manage the disease.

According to the American Cancer Society's *Cancer Statistics 2025* report, the cancer mortality rate in the United States has declined 34 percent from 1991 to 2022, averting roughly 4.5 million deaths. It is clear that cancer is less likely to kill you today than in the past. This trend is mostly due to more frequent and earlier detection, advances in treatments, and a significant decrease in tobacco use. The lung cancer death rate for men has dropped by 58 percent from 1990 to 2020, and by 36 percent for women from 2002 to 2020. Certain cancers have seen dramatic improvements in survival rates. The five-year survival rate for leukemia has more than doubled since 1975. In the 1970s, the overall cancer survival rate, meaning all cancers combined, was 49 percent. Today it is 70 percent.

Remission and survival rates on the whole show that people are not only living longer in remission but also living longer with their cancer being treated as a chronic condition. And now that health disparities are being quantified and tracked in ways they never used to be, people from underserved backgrounds, who are statistically more likely to suffer a poor outcome from cancer, will hopefully see greater and more personalized access to education and care. Because cancer biology is so complex, and many facets of it are still poorly understood, the most effective way to stop cancer still seems to be prevention. (See Question 27—What is the prognosis for someone diagnosed with cancer?)

30. How is a treatment plan created?

Once a patient is diagnosed with cancer, treatment planning begins. A treatment plan is a detailed and highly personalized strategy, a roadmap, created to manage the patient's care. It is developed using all the information gathered during the patient's assessment. It factors in the patient's age, health, medications and supplements, and any ongoing health problems that might affect the patient's ability to tolerate therapy. Prognostic factors such as diagnosis, cancer stage, and tumor grade will also inform the goals of the treatment. It includes recommended therapies, their timing and expected outcomes, and it is reevaluated whenever necessary.

The process of creating a treatment plan involves a multidisciplinary team whose recommendations are based on standard-of-care practices. The various specialists include the medical, surgical, and radiation oncologists who administer the therapies, radiologists, and pathologists to read and interpret findings, and nursing staff, counselors, and social workers who provide care and support. The specific type of cancer may require input from other medical experts like lung or liver specialists. The patient may also need support from pharmacists, physical therapists, or nutritionists to cope with the treatments' side effects.

When a treatment plan is complete, the patient will often have a teaching session with their doctor or care team during which the plan will be described step by step, and the patient will be educated on their particular therapies, how they work, how to manage side effects, and strategies for self-care.

Throughout the process, the most important thing is that the care provider or team communicates closely with the patient. Medical professionals who work in the field of oncology understand that a cancer diagnosis is shocking and overwhelming, and that there is a need for emotional support as well as medical expertise. The patient should be kept informed and actively participate in their own treatment decisions. It is just as important for the patient to communicate with their team what and how much they want to be told. Some people crave information about their cancer treatment and others would rather just know the minimum. Care providers do their best to accommodate the unique needs of each patient.

The patient's input is also critical with respect to their personal goals, values, lifestyle, and constraints. There may be more than one treatment option to weigh, or a second opinion to evaluate. Special considerations might include the mental and physical consequences of the treatment like stress, mobility, or fertility, its effect on their quality and quantity of life, its financial and insurance related implications, and even practical factors like transportation and lodging. Each patient must decide what they are willing to undertake. They should be encouraged to ask questions every step of the way.

Concerns, and "what-ifs" need to be addressed because no treatment plan is completely predictive, and the decision-making will be an ongoing process. Ultimately, the decision to accept or refuse treatment is with the patient. If they are an adult and able to make decisions, they will go through a process called informed consent. This agreement between the patient and the health care provider indicates they have been informed about the treatment and understand the information provided, and gives permission for care, treatment, or services. The patient also has the right to refuse part or all of the treatment.

The plan, which is discussed in person and shared in writing, will cover diagnosis and stage, specific test results, the recommended treatment along with schedule, dosing, and delivery, expected side effects and long-term effects, secondary treatments like pain management or oxygen, the role of the caregivers, resources for emotional and mental health support, advance directives like living wills or do-not-resuscitate orders, and treatment goals.

The treatment goal is, ideally, to achieve a cure, but sometimes the realistic goal is to increase survival time where there is no possible cure, or to increase quality of life without an increase in survival time. These goals all depend on the prognosis. The prognosis is the forecast or likely course of the disease. All cancer therapies have risks; they can be toxic, invasive, and injurious, in both the short and long term. So, the overall aim is that therapy should offer benefits that outweigh its risks. There is little point in curing the cancer if you cannot save the patient.

Treatment choices depend on the type of cancer and its aggressiveness. The most appropriate therapy will be whatever is most effective at removing, destroying, or stopping the disease. Local therapy is a treatment for localized cancer. It directly targets a visible, clearly defined tumor or other specific area of the body. The main types of local cancer therapy include surgical and ablative procedures, radiation therapy, and certain energy-based therapies like photodynamic therapy. These are all ways of physically removing or destroying a tumor. There is no local therapy option for blood cancers since they are usually considered systemic at diagnosis. Hodgkin lymphoma is an exception as it develops along a predictable path in the lymphatic system and is very susceptible to radiation.

A systemic therapy is a treatment that affects the entire system, and is usually the best option for metastatic disease because it reaches cancer cells anywhere in the body. All systemic therapies have some degree of side effects and toxicity because they circulate everywhere and will affect normal cells as well as cancer cells. The main types of systemic cancer therapies include chemotherapy, hormone therapy, immunotherapy, targeted therapy, and stem cell transplant. These are drugs or agents that are introduced through the bloodstream or ingested in pill form.

For most cancers, stage is the most important factor for predicting outcome. Most stage I cancers are treatable with local therapy alone. This means only the tumor needs to be addressed, usually with surgery. Sometimes stage II cancers are also treated with systemic therapy, like chemotherapy, because there is a chance the cancer has already spread. Stage III always requires systemic therapy for this reason, but has a less favorable prognosis. For stage IV cancers, local therapy is only used to help with immediate issues related to the tumor. Systemic treatments are necessary to address metastasis, but they tend to lose their effectiveness long-term, which is why stage IV disease generally has poor outcomes.

Cancer treatment plans can also be guided by genetic testing, to see if the patient has any inherited mutations that might dictate how the disease will progress. Treatment plans now often include molecular profiling, also known as biomarker testing, especially with patients who have metastatic cancer. Biomarkers are specific indicators, including genes or proteins that can be detected in the body or the tumor itself. This kind of testing examines DNA,

RNA, and proteins for more targeted or precision approaches to treatment. This personalized information can sometimes reveal whether or not their cancer will respond to certain drugs, thereby saving the patient from a trial-and-error approach.

Cancer treatment is often scheduled in phases. Treatment that is administered before surgery, to shrink a tumor, for example, is called neoadjuvant therapy. After surgery, adjuvant therapy is administered to eliminate any cancer cells that may remain in the system. Throughout the treatment, there are various kinds of monitoring and ongoing assessments. These include imaging and blood tests to track progress and detect signs of recurrence.

The schedule is also subject to the patient's response to the treatment. Sometimes patients want a break from treatment for personal reasons, or they just need relief from the side effects. Sometimes the medical care team will recommend a break because there are other health issues at play, or to perform certain tests. A break in treatment should always be a discussion between the patient and the cancer care team because timing and order in treatments can make a difference.

Patients are warned about side effects, and their medical team will advise them on self-care strategies to help them cope. Hydration is critical; not only does it help the body function, it addresses constipation, dry mouth, nausea, and fatigue. Activity is important; even walking and stretching can help with fatigue and improve well-being. Nausea is an issue with many cancer treatments, so keeping a good caloric intake is critical. Patients are advised to eat foods high in nutrients that are easy to chew and swallow. Cold treats and ice chips also help with nausea. Many treatments dry the skin, and some can make it sensitive to sunlight, so moisturizing and using sunscreen becomes very important. Some complementary therapies like acupuncture or massage provide a great deal of relief, and many patients find meditation and spiritual practices help alleviate stress. Good sleep is healing, for both the mind and body. Side effects should be carefully tracked and reported so they can be addressed as early as possible. Many of them can be managed and treated with additional medication and lifestyle changes.

Palliative care is specialized care aimed at managing symptoms and pain and improving quality of life. There has been a recent shift toward integrating palliative care earlier in the cancer treatment process and using it alongside curative or life-extending care. Studies show that patients receiving palliative care experience fewer hospitalizations, report a higher quality of life, and experience longer survival times.

In the case of cancer that has severe side effects, or is very advanced, inoperable, or otherwise not curable, the treatment plan may shift the focus to palliative care only. In this instance, the medical team may have an honest conversation with the patient about avoiding futile treatment, relieving pain, and finding emotional support.

31. How are tumors removed, and what are the potential side effects?

The most effective way to address a tumor is to completely remove or destroy it using surgery. Surgery is a standard and primary cancer treatment option. Throughout history, surgery has been a harrowing and dangerous option for patients, but with modern antiseptic surgical procedures, anesthesia, and antibiotics, it has become one of the most effective treatments for cancer. According to the University of Texas MD Anderson Cancer Center, almost 60 percent of cancer patients undergo some type of surgical procedure to treat their cancer.

Depending on the type of cancer, its stage, and its location, the goal of surgery is to remove as much cancer from the body as possible. The current emphasis is on tissue-conserving surgery, which removes detectable cancer without sacrificing any more healthy tissue than necessary. Studies show the outcomes are comparable to more extensive surgeries but are much less mutilating and debilitating. Surgery might be the only procedure required, or it might be used in conjunction with other types of treatments like adjuvant (presurgical) or neoadjuvant (post-surgical) chemotherapy or radiation. Surgery works most effectively with localized and early-stage solid tumors.

Surgical resection is the physical removal of a mass. It is used in diagnosing and staging cancer, for performing biopsies, and examining organs and lymph nodes. In the event that the entire tumor is eliminated, it can even be curative. If it is unsafe to remove the tumor completely, surgery is used to debulk it. This involves removing as much of the tumor as possible, sometimes doing so more than once. Surgery can be preventive in the case of removing tissue that is likely to develop into cancer. It is also used as a palliative treatment to relieve pain even if there is no cure. Surgery is often used to support other types of treatments, and it is used reconstructively to repair the ravages caused by more radical procedures. There are several kinds of surgical procedures that result in the removal or the destruction of the tumor.

Conventional or open surgery involves creating an incision through skin, tissue, sometimes bone, and removing all of the detectable tumor. The tumor's margin, which is the healthy tissue surrounding it, will also be removed. The surgeon will examine, and sometimes even remove the nearby lymph nodes. The advantage of open surgery is that it makes it easy for the surgeon to see and access the tumor. And with complete removal, the biological complexities of the tumor microenvironment that make it so hard to treat are simply not an issue. Surgical removal is the only treatment to which all the tumor's cells are equally susceptible.

The risks of open surgery are pain, infection, bleeding, scarring, or damage to surrounding tissues, organs, or nerves, and reaction to anesthesia. It can sometimes result in disfigurement or dysfunction. Open surgery is impossible if the tumor is inaccessible or located inside a vital organ. But it is an effective standard treatment for any localized cancer that can be accessed through an incision, including skin, breast, thyroid, head and neck, colorectal, kidney, and ovarian.

Minimally invasive surgery, also called laparoscopic or keyhole surgery, is a procedure that uses a few small incisions to introduce specialized tools and cameras, and the surgery is performed manually. Robotic surgery uses similar incisions through which the surgeon operates specialized optics and robotic arms to perform the surgery remotely. Some minimally invasive procedures like endoscopic and transoral surgeries do not require incisions but are performed through a natural body cavity, like the mouth, rectum, or vagina.

Because this kind of procedure uses much smaller incisions than open surgery, it offers faster recovery, less pain, and fewer complications. It sometimes does not even require general anesthesia. But the drawbacks are that this kind of surgery takes longer and can be very costly. It sometimes involves pumping gas into the abdominal cavity so the surgeon can see and access the organs better, which may increase the risk for patients with heart and lung conditions. Laparoscopic and robotic surgeries are commonly used to treat colorectal, prostate, kidney, liver, and bladder cancers, as well as some gynecological cancers.

Mohs surgery, also known as microscopically controlled surgery, is a technique in which thin layers of tissue are shaved off and examined one at a time under the microscope until no more cancer is detected. This procedure is used for certain skin cancers on the head or face, for example, where the extent of the cancer is unclear, but as much healthy tissue as possible needs to be preserved. This process, which allows the tissue to be rapidly analyzed during an ongoing surgical procedure, is called intraoperative pathology consultation. The tissue is rapidly frozen so that it can be thinly sliced, stained, and examined. The findings of the frozen section can then inform the surgeon's next move. In addition to Mohs surgery, intraoperative pathology consultation is used to diagnose masses, analyze tumor margins and lymph nodes, and address unanticipated findings.

Interventional radiology is the use of imaging technologies like x-rays, ultrasound, and MRI to guide specialized tools through the body. It combines radiology and surgery to help the surgeon get small instruments like catheters and needles directly to the tumor. Interventional radiology is used to guide tumor removal, biopsies, deliver chemotherapy, and embolization, which is a procedure that blocks the flow of blood to a tumor. Intraoperative fluorescence is another innovative approach to getting real-time imaging during surgery. It helps achieve complete tumor removal by using fluorescent dyes which selectively bind to the tumor. When the tissue is illuminated with a specific wavelength of light, it fluoresces, allowing the surgeon to operate more precisely.

Ablation is a way to destroy cancer cells without precise surgical dissection. Localized ablation is a kind of minimally invasive procedure that uses heat, extreme cold, and other energy sources to ablate, or destroy, cancerous tissue with targeted precision. It is a useful technique for areas of the body that are harder to access. Ablation is very effective for small, localized tumors and usually requires only local anesthesia. It also offers an alternative for patients who are not candidates for surgery due to their health because these procedures can often be performed on an outpatient basis.

Some ablation procedures use localized hyperthermia, or very high temperatures, to destroy cancer cells and nearby blood vessels. An image-guided probe is inserted into the tumor where the cells are heated. Radiofrequency ablation (RFA) uses a probe to heat the targeted tissue using an oscillating electrical current. It is the most common ablation procedure.

Laser surgery, sometimes called laser-induced thermal therapy (LITT) uses high-intensity light set to specific wavelengths in order to burn or kill tumor cells. It is often used to treat small tumors in the vagina, penis, lung, or skin. Microwave ablation uses heat generated with microwaves. Electrosurgery uses alternating electric current to cut, coagulate, or fuse tissue. Heat has the advantage of killing bacteria and sterilizing the wound, so these procedures result in less blood loss than surgery, have a lower risk of infection, and faster recovery time.

Cryoablation uses liquid nitrogen, argon gas, or a very cold probe to freeze cancer cells. It is used to treat surface cancers like skin cancer but can also be guided through a small incision into the body to deliver the frozen gas to an internal tumor. Percutaneous ethanol injection is an ablation technique that uses ethanol injected directly into the tumor which essentially dehydrates the tumor's cells. This procedure is generally used for small tumors in the liver, and sometimes for recurrent thyroid cancer.

These procedures can often be performed on an outpatient basis. Ablation is very effective for small, localized tumors and usually requires only local anesthesia. One of the drawbacks of ablation is that the procedure leaves no tissue behind to examine microscopically, and in some cases, the procedure needs to be repeated. Common risks include pain, infection, and potential damage to surrounding tissues. Ablation is most often used to treat tumors in the liver, kidney, lung, bone, adrenal gland, breast, pancreas, and thyroid, especially when the cancer has metastasized to these organs from elsewhere.

One of the misconceptions about cancer surgery is that cutting into the tumor will cause cancer to spread to other parts of the body. Although technically possible, this is very unlikely. Parathyroid and gallbladder tumors, and some sarcomas do have a low risk of cancer spread as a result of surgery, but this is extremely rare, and the benefits of the treatment far outweigh the small risk. In the past, when larger needles were more common in taking biopsy samples, the risk was higher, but modern biopsies are more likely to be performed using small needles, or by cutting through the skin to remove a piece of the tumor. Surgeons are increasingly likely to remove the entire tumor upfront, rather than just performing a preliminary biopsy, especially if it is likely to be cancer. Modern surgical procedures and imaging, as well as the extensive precautions taken by surgeons, ensure that these very small risks are minimized.

32. How does radiation work and what are the potential side effects?

Radiation therapy, also called radiotherapy, uses the high-energy waves of ionizing radiation to destroy cancer cells. Soon after the discovery of x-rays, scientists realized that radiation affected fast-growing cells in the body and began using it as a cancer treatment. Today, it is one of the most commonly used cancer therapies. According to the National Institutes of Health (NIH), around 50 percent of all cancer patients receive radiation therapy during the course of their treatment.

High-energy ionizing radiation can, in high doses, kill cancer cells. Radiation causes severe DNA damage, either directly and so severely that the cells die, or, more commonly, as a result of the reactive oxygen species (ROS) it produces inside the cell. This byproduct of cellular respiration activates cell cycle control checkpoints, which slows the division of rapidly proliferating cancer cells and causes some of them to die. It also slows down their ability to repopulate the tumor. The damage to the cancer cells is dose-dependent, so the therapeutic goal of radiation therapy is to deliver a total dose of radiation that will destroy all the cancer cells. However, the dangers of radiation are also dose-dependent, and the effects of radiation are cumulative. There is a lifetime limit to how much radiation healthy tissues can tolerate, which is why sometimes radiation therapy cannot be used again on the same part of the body. The course of therapy has to be carefully designed to minimize harm to normal cells and maximize harm to the tumor.

Radiation is generally used as a local therapy for localized or regional cancers. It must be focused enough to damage the cancer cells while causing minimal collateral damage to the surrounding healthy cells. It is used alone or in combination with surgery, and usually with the intent to cure. As a neoadjuvant (pre-surgical) treatment, it can be used to shrink a tumor. As an adjuvant (post-surgical) treatment, it can be used to eliminate any residual cancer cells. Radiation is rarely appropriate for metastatic cancers, except to relieve localized complications that might be disruptive or painful for the patient.

Radiation therapy is used to treat many types of cancer. Most often it is used to treat cancers of the head and neck, brain tumors, lung, prostate, and breast cancer, especially in their early stages. It is also used to prepare the body for bone marrow transplants.

There are two main ways of delivering radiation to a cancer patient and their use depends on the tumor's type, grade, and location, and the patient's ability to withstand the treatment and its side effects. These are external beam radiation (EBR) and brachytherapy.

External beam radiation (EBR), also called teletherapy, uses a radiation source from outside the body. EBR relies on deeply penetrating radiation and is the most common form of radiation therapy because it has multiple uses. It can be applied in complex or sensitive areas and precisely adjusted in real time.

The types of beams used in this therapy include photon, particle, electron, and proton beam radiation.

- Photon beam radiation uses high-energy x-rays to damage cancer cells. It is the most common type of radiation therapy.
- Particle beam radiation uses protons or neutrons that are released as a stream of high-energy particles. A particle beam can travel deep into the

body and delivers more radiation to the tumor while limiting the damage to the cells around it.

- Electron beam radiation does not penetrate as deeply into the body and tends to be used on surface cancers.
- Proton beam radiation typically causes less damage to normal tissue. It is used to treat tumors that are close to critical structures, such as the brain, eyes, spinal cord, and heart.

EBR can be directed in a variety of ways, including three-dimensional conformal radiation therapy, which delivers beams from different directions so as to match the shape of the tumor. Image-guided radiation therapy uses three-dimensional imaging to make precision adjustments. Intensity-modulated radiation therapy can adjust the strength of the beam so stronger doses can be directed into the tumor and damage to the surrounding tissue can be minimized. Stereotactic radiosurgery is usually used to treat brain tumors, as it delivers one large precision dose in a single treatment. Radiation can also be administered during surgery using intraoperative radiation therapy. This is useful in cases where the tumor cannot be completely removed and there is a high chance of recurrence.

EBR is used in early-stage cancers to destroy or shrink the tumor, to prevent cancer from returning somewhere else, and to treat various symptoms. It is a preferred treatment for localized, or isolated cancers like breast, colon, lung, prostate, and uterine.

Brachytherapy, or internal radiation therapy, uses a radiation source that is placed inside the body, close to or within the tumor. Brachytherapy consists of a radioactive isotope that has short-range penetration, usually delivered in beads, seeds, wires, or needles, which are implanted into the tumor. Sometimes radiation is delivered by a wand inserted into a natural body cavity. This is used to treat cancers of the head and neck, breast, cervix, prostate, and eye. Brachytherapy tends to be faster and more convenient, and it limits the damage to normal cells better than EBR, but it requires more invasive procedures to accomplish.

Sometimes, a radioactive drug is administered by mouth or intravenously. This is called systemic radiation. This form of radiation therapy uses radioactive drugs which travel through the bloodstream and attach to receptors on the tumor's surface. It is used to treat prostate, bone, and thyroid cancer. Because the entire body is potentially exposed to radiation, this is the riskiest type of radiation therapy.

The goal of radiation is not always to treat with the highest dose. Low-dose radiotherapy is sometimes used to trigger an immune response that might cause tumors to shrink or make them more responsive to other cancer treatments.

To deliver the maximum radiation with the minimum side effects, the treatment is split up into smaller doses spread out over time. These are called "fractions." Aside from making the treatment more tolerable, the technique of fractionation also exploits certain features of the cancer cells. The damage to healthy cells caused by the smaller dose is repaired in between treatments, but tumor cells are less efficient in repairing themselves. They lack the healthy cells' advantages and are less likely to survive after each treatment. Tumors that regenerate more quickly after a radiation treatment tend to be more resistant to the therapy, so the timing of delivering the fractions depends on how the tumor reacts. The goal is to injure the tumor repeatedly before it can regenerate.

Tumors are made up of complex cell populations that are genetically and metabolically diverse, so treatment like radiation will affect different parts of the tumor differently. As a result, patients can develop radiation resistance because the tumor cells have adapted to the changes in their environment.

Before radiation treatments begin, the radiation oncologist will schedule a planning session and simulation. During this process, the patient will be carefully and precisely positioned using lasers in order to determine the treatment field or area. The treatment field will be marked with semi-permanent dots. This ensures that every radiation treatment will be delivered in exactly the same way.

Sometimes this process requires physical restraints such as head masks and body molds. Having the treatment itself is similar to getting an x-ray, with heavy shields being used to protect the parts of the body that are not being treated. Patients generally receive treatment every day, five days a week, for five to eight weeks, with the total dose and timing depending on the size and location of the cancer, and the health of the patient. This type of therapy is, for the most part, an outpatient procedure.

Radiation therapy is an effective, flexible, sometimes curative, high-precision cancer treatment. But it has many short- and long-term side effects, including skin redness or irritation similar to sunburn, fatigue, pain, swelling, and discomfort. Depending on where the radiation is administered it may cause organ damage, difficulty swallowing and tooth decay, cough and shortness of breath, nausea, vomiting, and diarrhea. Long-term side effects include scarring in the treated tissues, nerve damage, heart or vascular issues, anemia, and infertility. The major drawbacks of radiation are the possibility of developing radiation resistance as repeated treatments become less and less effective, and the small but frightening risk of developing a second cancer. Radiation therapy also requires repeated, sometimes daily, travel to a treatment center with specialized equipment, making it physically taxing as well as disruptive. Patients with other health conditions might not be able to tolerate the treatment at all.

33. How does chemotherapy work and what are the potential side effects?

Chemotherapy, or chemo, is a type of cancer therapy that uses chemical-based drugs to stop or slow the growth of cancer cells, either by killing them or preventing them from dividing. The widespread use of chemotherapy began in the 1940s and it is the oldest and most commonly used type of cancer treatment, aside from surgery. According to the Dana-Farber Cancer Institute, more than half of all cancer patients will receive chemotherapy.

Chemotherapy is a systemic cancer therapy, meaning it is delivered to the entire body and affects both cancer and healthy cells. The drugs are most commonly introduced through the bloodstream by injection or infused directly into a vein or artery. They can be administered topically on the skin, or orally as pills, capsules, or liquid. They can also be introduced directly into the abdomen or even injected directly into the fluid around the spinal canal or near the brain.

The goal of chemotherapy is to destroy cancer cells, or to control their growth in the event they cannot be eliminated. It is also used to ease cancer symptoms. It can be used on its own as a primary treatment, especially in cases of metastatic and blood cancer. It is also used in conjunction with other drugs and therapies like radiation and immunotherapy to enhance their effectiveness. It can be administered before primary treatment, to shrink tumors before radiation therapy or surgery, and after primary treatment, to reduce the risk of the cancer returning.

Some chemotherapy drugs are cytostatic, meaning they stop the growth of highly proliferative cells without destroying them. But most chemotherapies are cytotoxic, or cell-killing drugs that are designed to destroy multiplying cells. These drugs bind to the DNA in the cells and stop them from being able to replicate. This class of drugs includes alkylating agents, platinum drugs, antimetabolites, topoisomerase inhibitors, antineoplastic antibiotics, and naturally occurring products like plant alkaloids.

- Alkylating agents induce breaks in the DNA, disrupting its structure and leading to cell death.
- Platinum drugs, or platins, bind directly to the DNA preventing replication and repair.
- Antimetabolites block cell division by replacing essential proteins and molecules during DNA synthesis and interfering with the cell cycle.
- Topoisomerase inhibitors prevent the enzyme that splits and rejoins strands of DNA from functioning.

- Antineoplastic antibiotics are types of molecules derived from living organisms that obstruct DNA replication.
- Plant alkaloids function as mitotic inhibitors, which means they block cells division by breaking the filaments which hold the chromosomes in place.

The choice of chemotherapy drug depends on the type of cancer, the overall health of the patient, and whether the patient has had chemotherapy before. Depending on how it is administered, patients receive chemotherapy during a hospital stay, in an outpatient setting like a doctor's office or clinic, or at home.

The most common way to administer chemotherapy is intravenously, through a catheter into a vein in the arm, or into a specially implanted device called a mediport or port-a-cath. This central venous catheter is surgically implanted under the skin, often in the chest or arm, and has a catheter which is connected to a large vein. Mediports are used with patients who need frequent treatments, transfusions, or blood draws, and allow for multiple therapies to be delivered at one time. Pumps are often attached to catheters and ports and can be carried externally or implanted under the skin surgically.

Treatment schedules can vary, but generally, patients receive chemotherapy in cycles. A cycle will consist of treatment followed by a period of rest during which the patient heals and builds up new healthy cells. For example, a two-week cycle would consist of treatment the first week followed by one week of rest. Missing a cycle is rarely recommended, but occasionally the care provider will advise a change in the schedule to accommodate the personal needs of the patient or manage their side effects.

Intravenous chemotherapy generally needs to be overseen by trained personnel in a special facility, and patients must practice some home safety measures to protect others from contact with their body fluids. All chemotherapy requires careful and regular monitoring because of its serious side effects and toxicities which can be debilitating or even lethal.

Chemotherapy is most commonly used to treat breast, lung, ovarian, pancreatic, and colorectal cancer, as well as leukemia and lymphoma. As treatment goes on, progress is tracked using physical examinations, imaging, and blood tests. The benefits of chemotherapy are that it can significantly reduce tumor size for easier surgical removal, eliminate microscopic cancer cells to prevent recurrence, and prolong survival.

But the downside of chemotherapy is that, like all systemic therapies, it has toxicities and adverse effects. It is nonspecific, meaning it impacts all rapidly dividing cells, including healthy ones. So, a significant aspect of chemotherapy treatment is monitoring and managing side effects. These may vary depending on the drug itself, the cancer, and the patients' overall health. Some patients have many side effects, and some have none at all. Most fade after chemotherapy is over, but some long-term effects can linger for months or years.

Short-term side effects include nausea and vomiting, anemia, fatigue, changes in appetite and weight, hair loss, changes in skin and nails, and an increased risk of infection. Long-term side effects can include damage to the heart, lungs, or kidneys. Damage to the reproductive organs can cause fertility issues. Peripheral neuropathy, which is damage to the nerves that results in pain, numbness, muscle weakness, and loss of balance, can last months or years and is sometimes permanent.

Managing side effects usually requires additional medications like anti-nausea drugs and lifestyle modifications including diet, exercise, stress relief like meditation, and rest, as well as psychological support like counseling and support groups. When side effects become too dangerous or disruptive, and when the benefits no longer outweigh the risks, the care team may decide to alter the dose or stop the therapy altogether.

Another drawback of chemotherapy, and other systemic therapies, is that they can create selective pressure for the cancer to become resistant to the treatment. There may be resistant cells that flourish once the other cells are destroyed, or the attack on the tumor will trigger mutations that can result in resistant cancer cells. The risk of treatment resistance highlights the importance of eliminating every trace of cancer, and with advanced disease, there is currently no way of knowing for sure if that has been achieved.

Combination therapies that combine chemotherapy with immunotherapies or targeted therapies are being used to increase effectiveness and reduce drug resistance. Advances in precision, or personalized medicine should also continue to increase the applications and reduce the side effects of chemotherapy.

34. How does hormone therapy work and what are the potential side effects?

Hormone therapy, also called endocrine therapy, is a cancer treatment that controls the progression of a hormone-sensitive tumor, not by destroying cancer cells but rather by stopping or slowing their growth. Hormone-sensitive tumors are types of cancers that rely on hormones like estrogen, progesterone, or testosterone to grow and spread.

This therapy is often used in combination with other therapies. It can act as a neoadjuvant therapy (to shrink a tumor before surgery or radiation), or as an adjuvant therapy (to lower the risk of the cancer returning). In more advanced cases, it can be used to slow cancer progression.

Hormones are produced by the endocrine system. They function as chemical messengers that travel all over the body to regulate metabolism, reproductive development, and growth. Some cancers are hormone-sensitive, or hormone-dependent, which means they have harnessed hormones to stimulate their own growth. They do this by activating the genes that produce hormone receptors, proteins on the surface of the cell that control a specific cellular activity, like growth and division. When cancer cells with these receptors bind to a hormone, they activate that cellular process.

Hormone-sensitive cancers are identified by testing tissue samples to see if they have estrogen receptors (ER), progesterone receptors (PR), or androgen receptors (AR). This test, called immunohistochemistry (IHC), reports the percentage of cells that are positive for hormone receptors. A positive result means the patient may benefit from hormone therapy. If the result is negative, hormone therapy is unlikely to be effective.

Hormone therapy drugs are taken orally or by injection. Each type works by either preventing the body from producing hormones, blocking hormones from attaching to cancer cells, or altering how hormones behave in the body.

Drugs that prevent the body from producing hormones work by chemically suppressing the production of hormones. They prevent the pituitary gland from making the hormones that stimulate the production of estrogen in the ovaries or testosterone in the testes. Aromatase inhibitors reduce levels of estrogen by reducing the function of the aromatase enzyme, which converts androgens into estrogens. CYP17 inhibitors are given to block the enzymes responsible for testosterone production, and progestins are given to suppress the production of estrogen. The body can also be prevented from producing hormones surgically, by removing hormone-producing organs. Removal of the ovaries (oophorectomy), or the testes (orchiectomy) can be an option that does not require any other long-term treatment, but it is irreversible.

Drugs that block hormones from attaching to cancer cells work by interfering with the hormone receptors. Androgen receptor inhibitors block testosterone from binding to androgen receptors in prostate cancer cells, and selective estrogen receptor modulators (SERMs) block the action of estrogen in certain tissues like breast tissue. Selective estrogen receptor degraders (SERDs) not only bind to estrogen receptors but also cause them to break down.

Drugs that alter how hormones behave in the body work by mimicking or modifying the action of hormones without necessarily preventing their production. These include progestins, which interfere with the effects of estrogen, anti-androgens which reduce the effects of testosterone, and corticosteroids which can alter hormone pathways in some cancers like leukemias, lymphomas, myeloma, and breast and prostate cancer. These steroids are also used to manage treatment side effects like pain, inflammation, and loss of appetite.

Hormone therapy is used to treat hormone-sensitive tumors in breast, endometrial, and prostate cancer. According to the National Cancer Institute (NCI), roughly 80 percent of breast cancers in women are ER positive. More than 50 percent are ER and PR positive. And although breast cancer in men is exceedingly rare, 90 percent of those cases are also ER positive. Between 80 and 90 percent of prostate cancers are androgen-dependent. Although hormone therapy is used to treat very few types of cancer, breast and prostate cancer are the most common cancers in women and men respectively, so it is a crucial intervention for many patients. Other cancers that may show hormone sensitivity are ovarian, thyroid, and certain lung cancers.

Hormone therapy is considered very effective in treating hormone-sensitive cancers and managing symptoms, and it significantly reduces the risk of cancer recurrence after the primary treatment. Sometimes the patient stays on the therapy for years after the primary treatment is over. And in some cases, hormone therapy can even be given preventively to women with a high risk of breast cancer.

The drawbacks of hormone therapy are that it alone does not cure cancer, and many cancers can become resistant to the therapy over time. The treatment also sometimes requires a long-term commitment that is hard for many to sustain.

Like all systemic treatments which circulate throughout the body, hormone therapies affect more than cancer cells. They also affect all the healthy cells that are responsive to hormones. This is significant because although hormones might fuel the progression of certain cancers, they also fulfill many protective functions in the body that are lost during therapy. The side effects of hormone therapy may include fatigue, nausea, bone loss and increased risk of fractures, hot flashes and night sweats, intimacy issues, and weight gain.

Women can experience vaginal dryness, mood swings, and increased risk of blood clots and stroke. Men can experience loss of libido, erectile dysfunction, muscle loss, weight gain, and breast tenderness or swelling. Long term, there is an increased risk of cardiovascular issues, bone fractures, depression, and anxiety. Hormone therapy can also temporarily or permanently disrupt hormone levels that are necessary for male and female fertility. Many of these side effects can be managed with lifestyle adjustments like diet and exercise, medications to strengthen bones and manage hot flashes, and counseling for depression.

35. How does immunotherapy work and what are the potential side effects?

Immunotherapy is a type of cancer treatment that boosts or harnesses the body's own immune system to recognize and destroy cancer cells. It is considered a revolutionary approach to cancer treatment because it is potentially more targeted, safer, and longer lasting than traditional treatments like chemotherapy.

Immunotherapy is a systemic therapy, meaning it affects the whole body at the same time, and it is a biologic therapy, meaning it is derived from living organisms. Precision, or personalized medicine, which tailors treatment to the patient's unique genetic profile and biomarkers, is central to immunotherapy and its ability to retrain the immune system. It is widely considered to be the fastest-growing field in cancer research.

The immune system protects the body against harmful invasion by pathogens like viruses, bacteria, and fungi. It is a complex network of tissues, organs, immune cells, and signaling molecules. The immune system works by recognizing threats, neutralizing them, and remembering them so it can respond faster in the future. It also has the very important ability to distinguish between threats that should be destroyed (kill) and the body's own healthy cells (do not kill). It does this by recognizing antigens, which are unique molecular markers. The antigens found on the surface of blood cells and body tissues identify them as "self." The antigens found on the surface of pathogens and abnormal cells identify them as "foreign."

The immune system has two main subsystems: the innate immune system and the adaptive immune system. The innate immune system is the first line of defense. It includes cells like natural killer cells and macrophages, which respond quickly and nonspecifically to an attack. Their response can trigger the adaptive immune system, which is the body's targeted defense against specific threats.

The adaptive immune system uses immune cells called B- and T-cells to respond to an attack. B-cells produce antibodies, and each type of antibody can recognize and target a specific abnormal or foreign antigen by attaching to its specific receptors on the surface of the targeted cell. T-cells target and destroy abnormal cells. Once these B- and T-cells are activated, some of them turn into memory cells which store information about the specific antigen and help mount a rapid antibody response if they encounter it again.

Given the effectiveness of the immune system, how does cancer manage to bypass and suppress its defenses? It is important to remember that cancer cells were once normal, healthy body "self" cells that the immune system recognized as "do not kill." It is an ability the cancer cells can harness. This is why the interplay between cancer and the immune system is an arms race.

The tumor can reprogram attacking immune cells to become tumor-promoting cells instead. Cancer cells take advantage of the innate immune system by initiating and exploiting inflammation. Inflammatory cells produce growth factors and cytokines, which are proteins that act as chemical messengers. Cytokines signal to the immune cells where to go and what to do, they can tell immature cells how to differentiate, and they can direct cells to multiply. Cancer cells subvert these cellular skills to promote their own growth and survival.

Cancer cells can also evade detection by the immune system. As healthy cells turn cancerous, they begin producing abnormal proteins that alert immune cells to their presence. Normally, this triggers an immune response that leads to the destruction of the affected cells. However, some cancer cells develop mutations that allow them to avoid this. These mutations help the cells hide their abnormal proteins or disable key parts of the immune response, essentially rendering them invisible to the body's defenses.

This process is known as cancer immunoediting and occurs in three phases: elimination, equilibrium, and escape. In the elimination phase, the immune system detects and destroys cancer cells. If some survive, they may enter the equilibrium phase in which they are held in check but not eliminated. These surviving cells tend to be more resistant to immune attack. Eventually, they may adapt and enter the escape phase, where they can evade the immune system entirely and begin to spread. When cancer is not fully eradicated, the immune system unintentionally puts evolutionary pressure on the cancer cells, forcing them to change and adapt. While the body is capable of destroying early-stage cancers, this gradual adaptation helps cancer cells survive and grow into larger, more dangerous tumors.

But immunotherapies can change the balance of power by helping the immune system in two ways; by boosting its tumor killing capacity, and by blocking the cancers cells' ability to undermine it. The basic categories of immunotherapy include immunomodulators, cancer vaccines, oncolytic virus therapy, monoclonal antibodies, immune checkpoint inhibitors, and adoptive cell therapy.

Immunomodulators are substances that can increase or decrease the immune response. With cancer, they are used to activate and excite immune activity. These nonspecific treatments interfere with the growth processes of cancer cells. Immunomodulators include:

- Bacillus Calmette-Guerin (BCG) is originally a vaccine for tuberculosis. It is a treatment used for bladder cancer that uses weakened or inactivated bacteria to stimulate the immune system. It is also used to prevent recurrence.
- Artificially synthesized cytokines like interleukins and interferons are used to enhance immune activity and act directly on the cancer to inhibit growth. This treatment is used in kidney cancer, melanoma, multiple myeloma, and some forms of leukemia.
- Immunomodulating drugs like thalidomide are used in cases of multiple myeloma to target immune pathways and inhibit inflammation, cell growth, and the production of new blood vessels.

Unlike preventive cancer vaccines, which are meant to prevent infections that may result in cancer, treatment vaccines are designed to be used therapeutically in people who already have cancer. Cancer vaccines stimulate the immune system to recognize and attack a specific cancer. Cancer cells have antigens called tumor-associated antigens, which are not present in normal cells. Treatment vaccines are used to "teach" the immune system to recognize and attack cancer cells that present that specific antigen.

Treatment vaccines can be produced using the patient's own immune cells, which are harvested and modified in a laboratory to respond to the tumor-associated antigen, and are then reinfused into the bloodstream. Vaccines can also be produced using the patient's whole tumor cells, peptides (small pieces of protein) from the tumor, or nucleic acids (bits of DNA or RNA) from the cancer cells. These personalized cancer treatment vaccines are currently used to treat prostate cancer and melanoma, but their expanded use is currently under development. Research is also underway to use vaccines to prevent cancer recurrence.

Oncolytic virus therapy is another type of vaccine used in immunotherapy. Oncolytic viruses are naturally occurring or genetically engineered viruses that can selectively infect and destroy cancer cells. Although the virus is capable of infecting healthy cells as well, these tend to successfully fight off the infection, whereas the cancer cells cannot. The virus is injected directly into the tumor and as it reproduces, it causes infected cancer cells to burst and die. The broken fragments of cancer cells trigger an additional body-wide immune response against the cancer. These oncolytic virus therapies are being used to treat melanoma and prostate cancer. Viruses called bacteriophages, which infect and kill bacteria, are currently being explored for their ability to carry therapeutic agents to cancer cells, and their potential to stimulate immune responses.

Monoclonal antibodies are used in immunotherapy to stimulate the immune system. Monoclonal antibodies are proteins cloned from a single laboratory-created antibody. They are designed to mimic natural antibodies by targeting and binding to specific antigens on the surface of cancer cells. Some monoclonal antibody therapies are considered targeted therapies because they target proteins or pathways to inhibit cancer growth. In immunotherapy, they are used to stimulate the immune system to find and destroy cancer cells directly.

Naked monoclonal antibodies are designed to bind to a cancer cell and "paint the target." This triggers an immune response, causing the cancer cell to be recognized and destroyed. They are called naked because they are unmodified.

Bispecific antibodies are designed to work in pairs so they can bind to two targets at once. One will attach to a cancer cell and the other will attach to an immune cell and the two will be drawn together, speeding up the immune response.

Immune checkpoint inhibitors are another type of monoclonal antibody which enhance the immune response by targeting specific checkpoints on T-cells. These checkpoints act as safeguards, preventing T-cells from attacking the body's own healthy "self" cells. T-cells have checkpoint proteins on their surface that scan for matching proteins on other cells, like checking for a password. When a matching protein is found on a "self" cell, it sends an "off" signal that deactivates the T-cell's killing response.

Under normal circumstances, this protects healthy cells from being targeted. However, some cancer cells exploit this system by producing the matching proteins, effectively "faking" the correct password. This tricks T-cells into shutting down, allowing the cancer to avoid destruction.

Immune checkpoint inhibitors work by blocking the interaction between the checkpoint proteins and their counterparts. By doing so, they prevent the "off" signal from being sent, keeping the T-cells active and able to attack cancer cells. Although response rates vary by cancer type, checkpoint inhibitors are approved for treating a range of cancers, including certain lung, kidney, breast, and colorectal cancers, as well as melanoma and Hodgkin lymphoma.

Adoptive cell therapy is a type of immunotherapy that uses the patient's own immune cells as "living drugs," by harvesting them, expanding or enhancing them, and then returning them to the bloodstream. It is a type of therapy that is customized for each individual patient. The process of growing and manipulating immune cells outside the body can take weeks to months. During this time, many patients are given other forms of treatment. Adoptive cell therapies include tumor-infiltrating lymphocyte (TIL) therapy, chimeric antigen receptor

T-cell (CAR T-cell) therapy, T-cell receptor (TCR) therapy, and dendritic cell (DC) therapy.

- Tumor-infiltrating lymphocyte (TIL) therapy uses immune cells called lymphocytes that have already penetrated the tumor. Although these cells are sensitized to the tumor and are capable of recognizing it, there may not be enough of them to overcome the tumor's immunosuppressive defenses. These lymphocytes are harvested, expanded, and multiplied, then reinfused into the patient. Sometimes the patient undergoes whole body irradiation ahead of time in order to eliminate competing immune cells. This type of immunotherapy is used to treat several cancers, including melanoma, lung, breast, and colorectal cancers. The process of removing specific immune cells and expanding, or growing them in large numbers outside the body before reinfusing them is also being used with cell killing T-cells and natural killer cells. This supercharges the immune system by boosting it with more of its own.
- Chimeric antigen receptor T-cell (CAR-T cell) therapy is the newest form of cell-based immunotherapy. It involves extracting T-cells from the patient and genetically engineering them to make a type of protein called a chimeric antigen receptor, which is a synthetic molecule that does not exist in nature. These receptors allow the T-cell to attach to their target proteins on the surface of cancer cells. These T cells are essentially personalized cancer killing machines. CAR-T cell therapy is being used to treat certain blood cancers and multiple myeloma. Treating solid tumors with CAR-T cell therapy has been less successful, as they present more substantial barriers to the T-cells. And solid tumors are made of many different kinds of cells, so targeting a single antigen means not all the tumor cells will be affected.
- T-cell receptor (TCR) therapy also involves genetically engineering a patient's T-cells. But unlike CAR T-cell therapy, which uses synthetic antibodies to recognize antigens on the *surface* of the cell, TCR therapy uses naturally occurring receptors that can also recognize antigens *inside* the tumor cell.
- Dendritic cell (DC) therapy uses altered dendritic cells to stimulate the immune system. Dendritic cells are immune cells that collect and present antigens to T-cells. They act like a "wanted poster" for the immune system. T-cells are then primed to seek out and destroy anything that has that antigen. In dendritic cell therapy, which is essentially a vaccine, dendritic cells are harvested, modified to display the targeted tumor's antigens, and returned to the patient. This therapy is used to treat some forms of prostate

cancer, as well as a rare and aggressive type of acute leukemia. The FDA has also granted fast-track designation to DC therapy for treating glioblastoma, a type of brain tumor, and pancreatic cancer.

Immunotherapy is generally considered more effective against "hot tumors," which are tumors that attract a strong immune response, because immune cells have already infiltrated the tumor. "Cold tumors" have very few immune cells present around or within them.

Immunotherapies can be administered in a variety of ways, usually intravenously at an infusion clinic, but also orally, applied topically to the skin, or injected directly into a specific body cavity, like the bladder.

Cancer cells are dynamic and diverse whereas most systemic drug therapies are fixed and uniform. This is the fundamental reason they have limited effectiveness against advanced cancers. But the immune system is ideally suited to fighting cancer because it has a variety of biological properties that help it adapt to cancer's complexity and ability to change. The immune system is systemic and can work anywhere in the body against any kind of cancer. It is also targeted as it can distinguish diseased cells from healthy ones. The immune system is not only adaptive, it also has memory, so it offers long-term protection.

This is why immunotherapy offers many exciting prospects. It is more targeted and specific than chemotherapy or radiation, so it also has fewer toxic side effects. It has been particularly effective with cancers that used to be considered virtually untreatable. In this respect, it can also provide an option for cancers that have not responded to other therapies. For a certain number of patients, immunotherapy drugs seem to be durable and sometimes even curative.

One of the current limitations of immunotherapy, however, is that it is successful only in a minority of patients, and predicting patient response is a huge challenge. According to Johns Hopkins Medical, the overall response rates are about 15 to 20 percent, which means most patients do not see the miracle cure that immunotherapy promises.

Not only are treatment failures common, but the therapy can also sometimes accelerate the disease instead, specifically with checkpoint inhibitors. The reasons for this are unclear and are a major focus of current research. In fact, how the immune system and cancer cells interact is still not fully understood. The FDA is currently investigating whether CAR T-cell therapies can cause secondary cancers, after several cases were observed in patients.

One reason for the unpredictable response to immunotherapies is that there are not enough biomarkers or obvious factors that indicate how well any given drug will work in any given individual. PD-1/PD-L1 expression, which is a protein that cancer cells use to switch off T-cells, is one of the few biomarkers being used at this time to determine whether or not immunotherapy is appropriate. Another marker, microsatellite instability (MSI), looks at the number of errors in short, repetitive DNA sequences. Tumor mutational burden (TMB) is a biomarker that reveals the total number of mutations across the tumor genome. Potential immunotherapy biomarkers are still being studied, including molecular markers from the tumor microenvironment and the gut microbiome.

Although based on the patient's own immune cells, many immunotherapies have some level of toxicity. Side effects can include autoimmunity and inflammation. Sometimes the patient experiences a release of cytokines called a cytokine storm. This side effect, known as chronic cytokine release syndrome (CRS), is, ironically, a sign that the body is responding to the therapy. It is typically managed with steroids, although in extreme cases it can be fatal.

Common side effects of immunotherapy include fever, chills, nausea and vomiting, low blood pressure, and fatigue. Serious side effects include neurological effects like confusion, seizures, and impaired speech.

Cost is another, considerable, downside to immunotherapy drugs. Insurance coverage varies, but these medications often cost around $100,000 per year, with one reaching costs of up to $1 million per year. One reason for this is that immunotherapy drugs usually involve a high level of personalization, including genetic testing and the production of unique cellular products, a time-consuming process in a specialized laboratory which can take weeks to months.

Drug resistance is always a factor in cancer treatments because cancers are so prone to mutation. Cancer cells can become resistant to immunotherapy when a new mutation stops them from expressing the antigen that is being targeted. The tumor microenvironment is quite hostile to immune cells and can eventually build physical and molecular barriers that prevent the treatment from reaching the cancer cells. Using drugs in combination, either by using multiple immunotherapies or by pairing them with other treatments like chemotherapy or radiation, can sometimes counteract resistance and reduce side effects.

36. How does a stem cell or bone marrow transplant work and what are the potential side effects?

A stem cell, or bone marrow, transplant is a procedure that replaces damaged or diseased blood-forming cells with healthy ones to help the body make new cells. Stem cell transplants are used to treat cancers that affect the blood, such as leukemia, lymphoma, and multiple myeloma.

Blood cells come from hematopoietic, or blood-forming, stem cells, within the bone marrow. They differentiate into red blood cells, white blood cells, and platelets. In blood cancers, these cells develop mutations and start producing abnormal, non-functioning blood cells which eventually crowd out the healthy ones.

Historically, stem cells were harvested from bone marrow; however, today it is much more common to harvest them from the bloodstream. Stem cells can also be harvested from the umbilical cord, in the case of a cord blood transplant. A stem cell transplant is a systemic therapy, meaning it affects the entire body at once.

The transplant procedure involves high doses of chemotherapy, and sometimes total body irradiation, to wipe out the abnormal and non-functioning blood cells. The infusion of new, healthy stem cells replaces the cells destroyed by the treatment and restarts the process of producing blood cells in the bone marrow.

The first stage of a stem cell transplant involves testing. Testing and evaluating the patient to see if they are healthy enough to undergo the treatment, and testing to find a matched donor, depending on the type of transplant. These tests involve scans, biopsies, and blood tests. Patients will often need some type of central venous catheter implanted under the skin to use during stem cell collection and infusion.

Whether they come from the patient or the donor, stem cells are collected from either bone marrow or the bloodstream. Bone marrow is harvested under general anesthesia, usually from the hip bone. It is a long procedure during which one to two liters of marrow are collected. The actual volume depends on the donor's body size and the host's requirements, but the focus is the concentration of stem cells within that volume. The donor's body will slowly regrow these cells within a few weeks. The harvested bone marrow is then processed to isolate the stem cells.

When transplant stem cells are harvested from the bloodstream, the donor is given a drug that promotes the production of stem cells. The blood is collected through a catheter and processed to isolate the stem cells, which are then preserved. The remaining blood is returned to the donor. This process, called apheresis, is an outpatient procedure that is repeated until enough stem cells have been collected. Sometimes the transplant is performed directly after collection, sometimes the stem cells are treated and frozen.

The conditioning treatment, which is also called myeloablation, is the pre-transplant treatment that destroys the remaining cancer cells in the body. It also suppresses the immune system to reduce the risk of rejection and allows for the newly transplanted cells to move to the bone marrow. Conditioning usually consists of high-dose chemotherapy, radiation, or sometimes both. Transplant procedures are usually performed in a hospital or specialized transplant center, often in rooms with special air filters and protective barriers to lower the risk of infection. The entire transplant procedure entails a long hospital stay, often several weeks or more throughout the process of the transplant and well into recovery.

The type of conditioning treatment depends on the type of cancer, the type of transplant, and any past cancer treatments. Chemotherapy will be administered either through the implanted central venous catheter or orally. If the treatment requires radiation, total body radiation is performed, in a single session or over the course of a few days. Conditioning is considered the point of no return, once conditioning treatment is done, the body will lose its ability to fight infection and make blood cells.

Transplanting the stem cells is done by infusion, like receiving a blood transfusion. The procedure can take several hours.

Recovery can take several months to a year. Engraftment, the process by which transplanted cells successfully "take" in the bone marrow, usually happens within the first thirty days after the transplant. While the transplant takes effect, the patient will be checked to see if their red blood cells, white blood cells, and platelets are increasing.

It takes much longer for the immune system to recover, however, months to years, depending on the type of transplant, so extra precautions are taken to avoid exposure to germs. In the weeks after, the immune system will be very weak. Patients are extremely susceptible to infection and are given a variety of antibiotics. If the patient received donor cells, they are also given anti-rejection drugs. Recovery can also be isolating and requires a lot of emotional adjustment. The process is not over once the patient is discharged. Once they are sent home, patients may need daily or weekly tests, examinations, and additional transfusions.

There are two main types of stem cell transplants, allogeneic and autologous.

An allogeneic transplant uses stem cells from a donor. The best donors tend to be siblings or other close family members, but a close match can also be found in someone not related, through a volunteer donor registry. These matches tend to be riskier but can still be lifesaving.

Stem cell donors are matched by examining markers called human leukocyte antigens (HLAs). Blood tests of the patient and potential donor determine if there is a match. If the match is not ideal, there is a higher risk of rejection. People inherit half of their HLA markers from their father and half from their mother, so the ideal donor is a sibling who has inherited the same markers. But the chance of having the same HLA types as a sibling is one in four. In looking for an unrelated donor, doctors will try to match all ten or twelve HLA markers in order to reduce the risk of rejection. Patients who do not have a close match may resort to a half-match. A biological parent will always be a half-match for their child, and in many cases a first degree relative can be as well. This increases the number of potential donors. Transplant teams are getting better at determining which mismatches can be tolerated, and which medications following the transplant will lower the risk of rejection.

Stem cells are collected from the donor and stored. After the conditioning treatment, the donor cells are infused. In some cases, depending on the specific cancer and the patient's immune system, the transplant may start destroying the cancer directly. This is called the graft-versus-malignancy or graft-versus-cancer effect. It happens when the donor immune cells see the remaining cancer in the patient as foreign and attack it. Allogeneic transplants are used to treat certain leukemias, lymphomas, multiple myeloma, myelodysplastic syndromes, and other bone disorders.

Blood from a newborn's umbilical cord can also be used for an allogeneic transplant, especially for patients without a well-matched donor. Cord blood contains a high number of stem cells. Collecting it poses no risk to the infant or mother, many new parents opting to donate cord blood to a public bank, or store it in a private bank in case it is needed some day. It is collected, processed, and stored immediately after birth. This means finding a donor match and moving ahead with cord blood is faster because it is already banked and available. A cord blood transplant is also less likely to be rejected, but it takes more time to engraft, leaving the patient vulnerable to infection for longer.

For patients whose age or health makes it dangerous to do a regular allogeneic transplant, there is a procedure called a mini transplant. This is also known as a non-myeloablative transplant or reduced-intensity conditioning. The patient receives lower doses of chemotherapy or radiation, with the goal of killing some cancer cells and some bone marrow but not all. The donor cells and the patient cells will exist in the body together until the donor cells take over the bone marrow. These new cells can then mount an immune response against the cancer.

The main benefit of an allogeneic transplant is the graft-versus-tumor effect, as well as the fact that the donor can always donate more stem cells if needed. The risks, however, are that the graft might not "take," and the donor stem cells could die or be destroyed by the patient's body before reaching the bone marrow. This is the reason allogeneic transplants have a much longer recovery time. The biggest concern is that the patient might develop graft-versus-host disease (GVHD), in which immune cells from the transplant donor attack the host. It can be acute (short-term) or chronic (long-term), and can cause many symptoms like rashes and burning, nausea, and weight loss. If it becomes a long-term issue, GVHD can potentially cause pain and bloating, blockages in the airways, and serious organ damage. GVHD reactions are common and are usually treated with steroids or other drugs to suppress the immune system. The closer the match, the less likely GVHD is to happen.

An autologous transplant uses the patient's own stem cells, which are collected and stored frozen, then reinfused after the conditioning treatment. Aside from blood cancers, autologous stem cell transplants are also used to treat other cancers like neuroblastoma, testicular, and certain pediatric cancers. Some patients receive a tandem, or double autologous, transplant, which means the transplant process is split into two courses of conditioning and two reinfusions, usually six months apart.

The main advantage of an autologous transplant is that the body is receiving its own cells back, which means there is no risk of rejection, and no risk of GVHD. The flip side of this benefit is that there is no chance of having a graft-versus-tumor effect because there is no immune mismatch. It is possible that the graft may fail, but this is less common. One of the biggest concerns with an autologous transplant is the risk that some cancer cells may have been collected along with the stem cells. Although the cells are rigorously processed and screened to prevent this, there is a potential risk that reinfusing them could reintroduce cancer and lead to a relapse.

The success rates for stem cell transplants vary widely depending on the type of cancer, the patient's age and overall health, the source of the stem cells, and degree of matching between donor and host. It does offer an overall higher potential for long-term remission or cure than other cancer therapies alone, particularly in cancer that has returned, or resisted therapy.

But all transplants come with serious risks and side effects. Regardless of the type of transplant, one of the most common side effects is infection due to a weakened immune system. Patients are usually required to take antibiotics for weeks to months after the transplant. Bone marrow suppression and bleeding are also an issue until the new graft begins producing blood cells, requiring additional blood and platelet transfusions.

Many side effects of stem cell transplants, like nausea and vomiting, are the result of chemotherapy or radiation. Mouth sores are another common side effect and occur when the linings of the mouth and gastrointestinal tract become inflamed. Long-term side effects include cataracts, hormone changes, organ damage, and infertility. There is also an increased risk of developing a second cancer, especially in patients who receive total body irradiation.

37. How does targeted therapy work and what are the potential side effects?

Targeted therapy is a treatment that attacks cancer by directly targeting the specific genes, proteins, and pathways that make cancer cells grow and spread. These drugs are directed at carefully identified molecular targets on, or inside, cancer cells, which minimizes the damage to healthy cells.

Targeted therapy is a type of systemic cancer treatment, which means it is circulated all over the body and affects the entire system. It is also a type of precision, or personalized medicine, which is a medical approach that is based on the patient's unique genetic profile and biomarkers.

These therapies work differently, depending on the specific feature they are targeting. They function by changing the cancer cells' proteins causing them to stop dividing and even die; by stopping the signals that form blood vessels and cutting off blood flow to the tumor; by making cancer cells more vulnerable to the immune system; and by delivering cancer killing drugs directly to the tumor.

Mutations in a cell's DNA can affect certain proteins related to cell growth, causing cells to multiply uncontrollably and develop into tumors. These proteins and their mutations are easier to target when they become more concentrated in the tumor cells than in the healthy cells around them, or when they undergo changes that make them distinct from other cells. Targeted therapy drugs are designed to interfere with these proteins and their growth-promoting signals.

There are two types of targeted therapy drugs, small molecule drugs and monoclonal antibodies.

Small molecule drugs tend to be chemical agents that are small enough to enter cells and bind to their target on the inside. Once there, the drugs mimic or block the target's function like a lock and key. The drug fits the lock which shuts down the function of the protein. Small molecule drugs typically end in "ib," like imatinib (Gleevec), indicating the drug is meant to inhibit a specific protein. They are usually administered orally with capsules or tablets.

Monoclonal antibodies are proteins cloned from a single laboratory-created antibody. Monoclonal antibodies are too large to penetrate the cell and instead attack targets on or around the surface.

Antibodies are produced by the immune system, and each type of antibody targets a specific abnormal or foreign substance known as an antigen. Antigens are found on bacteria, viruses, toxins, and your own body's cells—including cancer cells. Antibodies target specific antigens by attaching to their respective receptors on the surface of a cell. Generally, an antibody is only effective against a single specific antigen.

Monoclonal antibodies are used in immunotherapy to boost the immune system and block the way cancer cells get around it. But they can have many other functions and targets. By targeting specific proteins, monoclonal antibodies can be designed to disrupt cellular function, neutralize a toxin, and make cells clump together. Monoclonal antibodies called antibody drug conjugates (ADC) are engineered to transport and bind cancer treatments directly to the tumor, by delivering a toxic agent or a radioactive molecule.

Signal transduction inhibitors, which block the signals that tell cells to proliferate, are the most common targeted therapy drugs. Angiogenesis inhibitors block the growth of blood vessels that supply the tumor. Gene expression modulators change the way genes are expressed in the cancer cells. Apoptosis inducers cause the cancer cells to undergo programmed cell death.

Drugs that are monoclonal antibodies typically end in "mab," like trastuzumab (Herceptin). They are usually given intravenously by infusion like chemotherapy, in an outpatient setting like a doctor's office or clinic.

Targeted therapy drugs show a clear benefit for some cancer types such as breast, colorectal, lung, pancreatic, lymphoma, leukemia, and multiple myeloma, especially in combination with standard therapies. But because these drugs are targeted, they do not work on all types of cancer, nor do they work on all cancers of the same type. In order to work, the molecular target has to be present in the tumor, and it has to be active in driving its development, otherwise it will have little effect. So, prescribing a targeted therapy drug usually requires additional diagnostic tests like biomarker testing and genetic sequencing of the tumor to determine whether it has molecular features that can be targeted.

For example, breast cancers are routinely tested for certain biomarkers. Some of these cancers are identified as HER2 positive breast cancers because they overproduce a growth-promoting protein called human epidermal growth factor receptor 2 (HER2). The aggressive growth and spread of HER2 positive breast cancers are driven by this particular protein. The monoclonal antibody tratuzumab works by binding to the HER2 protein receptors on the surface of the cancer cells, stopping growth and slowing the cancer's progression. This drug would be ineffective against a cancer that did not have these particular protein receptors.

Other genetic mutations that can be treated with targeted therapy include BRCA1 and BRCA2 mutations which are often present in breast, ovarian, and prostate cancer, EGFR mutations which are found in some lung cancers, KRAS mutations which can appear in lung, colorectal and pancreatic cancer, and BRAF mutations which occur in around 50 percent of melanomas.

Sometimes, a gene that is driving cancer development is switched on or off rather than mutated. This change in the way the gene is expressed is called an epigenetic change. Because it does not affect the actual DNA sequence, it is reversible. This makes epigenetic changes good targets for therapy. Epigenetic therapies target the signals that control gene expression, resetting them so the genes are restored to their normal function. Epigenetic therapy is being used to treat some blood cancers, but it is also being studied for its potential to provide biomarkers for cancer diagnosis.

Targeted therapies are sometimes used as the primary treatment for certain cancers, but more often they are given in conjunction with other cancer treatments like surgery, chemotherapy, radiation, and hormone therapy. Targeted therapy can be used as a neoadjuvant treatment, to help shrink a tumor before surgery, or as an adjuvant treatment, to target any remaining cancer cells and help prevent recurrence. Some drugs are taken for a prescribed period, or until the cancer is gone. Others can be taken for the rest of your life, as long as the drug is tolerated or until it stops working.

The biggest advantage of targeted therapy is that it is a more precise treatment with fewer adverse effects than chemotherapy, which is nonspecific and highly toxic. But although targeted therapies are usually better tolerated, they do still come with their own side effects. These include issues with wound healing, high blood pressure, fatigue, mouth sores, rashes, dry skin, sun sensitivity, diarrhea and other gastrointestinal symptoms, changes in nail growth, and hand and foot syndrome (a painful redness and blisters that appear on the palms and soles of the feet). Other rare but more serious side effects include organ damage, autoimmune reactions, and the formation of holes in the walls of the gastrointestinal tract. Not everyone experiences side effects and those who do may experience them to varying degrees. Most side effects go away after the treatment is over, but this kind of therapy is relatively new among cancer treatments, and in many cases the long-term side effects are still unknown.

Targeted therapies have turned some serious cancers into treatable diseases. Cancers which were traditionally associated with a poor prognosis, like chronic myeloid leukemia (CML), are now associated with long-term survival. Targeted therapy works particularly well in CML because the disease is almost always caused by the same mutation. In contrast many other cancers are driven by multiple interacting factors, making it harder to find a single effective target.

This is why one of the biggest drawbacks of targeted therapies is drug resistance. Tumors are heterogeneous, meaning they are made up of many different types of cells with many different mutations driving their development. Because of this, going after a single target means it is unlikely the therapy will be effective against every cell in the tumor. As it eliminates the targeted cells, the treatment could start encouraging the proliferation of other, therapy-resistant cells. Or the cancer cells might produce new mutations in order to get around the action of the drug. (See Question 6—What is a tumor?)

Another drawback of these drugs is the price. Targeted therapies can cost tens of thousands of dollars per month, depending on the type of medication and how and where it is given to you. This reflects the cost of research and development, manufacturing, and market pressures.

38. How does photodynamic therapy work and what are the potential side effects?

Photodynamic therapy is a local, two-stage, minimally invasive procedure that involves administering a drug and then activating it using light. This standard treatment option for specific and localized cancer is an energy-based treatment, a form of ablation which minimizes the harm to healthy tissue. Although this therapy has been around for a long time, it is uncommon and specialized. It is considered a good option for patients who cannot tolerate more aggressive treatments.

Photosensitizers, or photosensitizing agents, are drugs that are completely inactive until they are exposed to a specific wavelength of light. The drug is applied topically or injected so that it penetrates the tissue. After the drug is given, there is a waiting period ranging from a few hours to several days, so that normal cells can metabolize and excrete it. Cancer cells, which hold on to the drug longer, are then exposed to a laser light which activates the drug.

This allows the cancer cells to be selectively targeted. Depending on where the tumor is, light is either applied directly, or it is inserted into a body cavity using an endoscope and a fiber optic cable. When activated, the drug interacts with oxygen in the tissues to produce highly toxic reactive oxygen species (ROS) which destroy the cells. The therapy is also used to damage blood vessels supplying the tumor or trigger an immune response against the tumor.

It is remarkably effective in the treatment of surface cancers, tumors that are on or just under the skin, and tumors near the linings of internal organs or cavities like esophageal cancer, or non-small cell lung cancer. Extracorporeal photopheresis (ECP), or photochemotherapy, is a kind of photodynamic therapy that is used to treat cutaneous T-cell lymphoma, and to reduce rejection after stem cell transplants. This blood-filtering procedure treats the patient's blood with a photosensitizing agent, exposes it to light, then returns it to the patient's body.

Because the drug is safe until it is activated, there are relatively few side effects. These include light sensitivity, swelling, and pain. The treatment is quick, has no long-term side effects, and can be performed multiple times. One of the drawbacks of photodynamic therapy is that it can only be used in areas where the light can reach. It is hard to focus laser light very deep into tissue, it cannot penetrate deeper than 1 cm, so the therapy is ineffective against deeper or larger tumors. Research is ongoing in making these types of drugs more powerful, in activating them with light that penetrates deeper into the tissue or activating them using other stimuli such as ultrasound. Clinical trials are ongoing to expand the use of photodynamic therapy to cancers in the brain, skin, prostate, cervix, and peritoneal cavity.

39. What are current cutting-edge cancer treatments?

Today, the field of oncology is evolving fast. Cutting-edge cancer therapies include a variety of innovative treatments, some of which are already in use, some of which are still in clinical trials at the time of publication. To be considered standard of care, these technologies and methodologies must be based on robust research, and they must have the potential to make a significant difference in patient outcomes. Many of these advances are a result of new developments in genetics and immunology, which have directed the shift toward precision medicine.

Precision, or personalized, medicine is a new approach that tailors treatment based on the unique molecular and genetic characteristics of both the patient and the cancer. It is considered to be the fastest-growing field in oncology.

Because tumor cells within the same type of cancer, and even within the same tumor, can vary genetically, this approach aims to improve outcomes by targeting the unique features of each tumor. Instead of a one-size-fits-all approach, precision medicine first identifies the targets in the tumor, then addresses them, improving effectiveness, reducing side effects, and avoiding the potential harm and wasted time of a futile treatment. Precision medicine advances the idea of tumor-agnostic therapy, a treatment that can address cancer based on its molecular features without regard to type or site of origin. The Food and Drug Administration (FDA) is beginning to approve new cancer drugs on this basis.

Next-generation DNA sequencing allows for millions of DNA strands to be sequenced simultaneously, making the process faster and cheaper than ever before. Sequencing the DNA of a tumor, or tumor profiling, is revolutionizing research into cancer treatments by allowing scientists to identify actionable mutations, specific features in the cancer cells that could be exploited.

This has led to adoptive cell therapies for the treatment of cancer, in which immune cells, which are drawn from the patient, are reengineered to target tumor cells and/or multiplied before being returned to the bloodstream. These therapies have seen some success in certain blood cancers and multiple myeloma, but they have been less successful at treating solid tumors, however, and factors like safety, effectiveness, and availability have presented challenges.

The Signatera Test, which has received Breakthrough Device Designations from the FDA, is a personalized blood test used to monitor and detect cancer recurrence in people who have already been treated for cancer. It is custom made for each patient by using a sample of their original tumor to detect tiny traces of circulating tumor DNA in their bloodstream. This helps doctors decide whether a patient needs additional treatment, like chemotherapy, after surgery. The goal is to avoid unnecessary treatment for those who do not need it, while catching hidden disease early in those who do. International guidelines are evolving to incorporate DNA sequencing as an essential step in clinical settings, enabling a more personalized way to treat the disease.

Gene editing can help develop more precise targeted therapies. CRISPR-Cas9 is a gene-editing tool that allows scientists to precisely cut and modify DNA. It is being studied as a way to create more effective cancer treatments by repairing faulty genes and enhancing immune cells. Gene editing has the exciting potential for direct cancer correction, such as replacing or restoring functional tumor suppressor genes, to help control cancer growth. (See Question 4—What role does mutation play in cancer development?)

The goal is to produce therapies that are more robust and stable, as well as creating an "off-the-shelf" product, using donor cells. These would be compatible with any patient, thereby avoiding the time and expense of producing each therapy individually, from the patient's own cells. Although this is a promising field, and the FDA has approved a CRISPR-based gene therapy to treat sickle cell disease, it has yet to be integrated into standard cancer care. Many CRISPR-based therapies are still in clinical trials at the time of publication.

CAR T-cell and other immunotherapies are evolving in other ways too. In order to get around the immune-suppressing barrier presented by the tumor microenvironment, scientists have developed "armored" CAR T-cells, which secrete proteins, like cytokines, effectively arming them to enhance their tumor killing abilities. Reversing the tumor microenvironment's ability to suppress immune responses remains a significant challenge for immunotherapies. Immune checkpoint inhibitors, which are monoclonal antibodies that override the mechanisms cancer uses to evade the immune system, are also seeing new developments. Clinical trials are testing drugs that target more inhibitory pathways, expanding their use against solid tumors.

A significant limitation of this kind of therapy is that customizing treatments using the patient's immune cells is time-consuming and costly. Allogeneic CAR T-cell therapies, which are an off-the-shelf version that uses T-cells from a healthy donor, are currently being evaluated. Another limitation is that this kind of therapy is successful only in a minority of patients, and predicting patient response is a huge challenge.

Next-generation immunotherapy research is also exploring more ways to activate the innate immune system against cancer cells, by harnessing natural killer (NK) cells and macrophages. These therapies, which are in early development or undergoing clinical trials, are designed to either boost the body's immune response, or target and neutralize the cancer cells' defenses.

RNA-based therapies are being developed which offer more targeted ways to fight cancer by modifying gene expression. Ribonucleic acid (RNA) is a molecule that takes a template of the cell's DNA and carries it elsewhere in the cell to build proteins. Because it is designed to carry information, RNA can be used to block or silence harmful genes. It can also train the immune system to target cancer cells by "reinterpreting" the DNA instructions. RNA interference therapies use RNA to silence the cancer-causing genes, which stop the tumor from growing. They make use of a synthetic strand of DNA to bind to the RNA in cancer cells, degrading or inhibiting it, and stopping the cancer cells from producing harmful proteins.

Messenger RNA (mRNA) vaccine technology, which has seen so much promise with infectious diseases, is now being engineered to fight cancer. An mRNA cancer vaccine is a personalized treatment that is designed to carry the instructions for specific proteins found in a patient's tumor. When the cells produce this protein, the immune system is trained to recognize and attack the cancer cells by producing the appropriate antibodies. Dozens of mRNA vaccines are in clinical trials, with approval for some expected by 2029.

These approaches do have side effects and risks. The most common vectors, or vehicles, for getting a given therapy to the cells are viruses. Risks include unpredictable immune responses, targeting the wrong cells, infection caused by the virus, and unanticipated errors in the genes. Research is ongoing to test other possible vectors such as stem cells and liposomes, which are tiny fat-based bubbles, as well as bacteriophages, which are bacteria-eating viruses that are not harmful to human cells.

Exosomes have gained attention for their possible therapeutic applications. Exosomes are extracellular vesicles, tiny bubble-like structures released by the cell, which carry molecules like proteins and RNA to communicate with other cells. They are likely to be useful in the early detection of cancer because cancer cells release exosomes with unique markers. They can also be used to carry anti-cancer drugs directly to the tumors. They offer the potential of becoming a more targeted and less toxic cancer therapy.

But they still present risks including toxicity, unwanted immune responses, and malignant transformation, which is the risk that normal cells could become malignant. Some clinics have marketed exosome treatments and even offered them to patients, but not only are the treatments not approved by the FDA, it has issued a consumer alert about the potential risks of these unregulated therapies. Exosome-based therapy is a promising tool in fighting cancer, but it is still in its initial stages, and more research is needed before it can overcome its regulatory issues.

Nanotechnology is another cutting-edge approach to cancer care. It is mainly used for improving drug delivery, enhancing imaging, and boosting immunotherapy. Developing an effective drug is one thing but getting it to the target presents a different set of challenges. The drug could either be degraded by the immune system before it reaches the target or be deflected by the tumor microenvironment once it gets there. While nanoparticles are small enough to pass easily through cells membranes, they are also large enough to contain a payload of therapeutic agents. And their larger surface can be tailored to target specific receptors on cancer cells. Wrapping a drug in nanoparticles and delivering it to the tumor also reduce systemic side effects because the nanoparticle prevents the drug from harming healthy cells. This technique can also be used to deliver vaccines and other immunotherapies. The FDA has approved several nanoparticle treatments and many more are in development. Liposomes and polymer-based nanoparticles are currently approved to deliver encapsulated chemotherapy in breast, pancreatic, and ovarian cancer.

Nanotechnology is also allowing for advances in targeted therapies such as photodynamic therapy, by improving the delivery and targeting of the photosensitizing drugs. Using a similar principle, in which light is used to trigger an anti-cancer reaction in the cells, nanoparticles are now being studied in the context of photothermal therapy. In photothermal therapy, near infrared light is applied after light absorbing nanoparticles have been delivered to the tumor. These nanoparticles are made of substances which convert light energy to heat when exposed to a specific light wavelength. Once exposed to this light, the nanoparticles heat up and destroy the cancer cells. This technique is minimally invasive, very precise, and could be combined with the delivery of other cancer therapies like chemotherapy.

Another cutting-edge form of nanotechnology that uses both physical and biological mechanisms is the molecular jackhammer. The molecular jackhammer uses an advanced organic molecule, a dye that binds to cancer cells and destroys them mechanically when it is activated. This noninvasive therapy consists of injecting molecular jackhammers near the tumor and exposing them to near infrared light, which triggers rapid vibrations in the molecule, generating forces that are powerful enough to break apart the cancer cells and induce cell death. This type of treatment minimizes side effects and collateral damage to healthy cells, and cancer cells are unlikely to be able to develop any resistance to it. The technology has performed well in treating melanoma in preclinical trials. The next step in testing is to see how effective it is against other forms of cancer.

Most research in nanotechnology is still ongoing because there are some challenges to overcome. Nanoparticles can cause toxicity if they accumulate in organs, the immune system may recognize them as foreign, and there is always a risk that they go off-target and harm healthy cells. Since this technology is relatively new, long-term side effects are still being studied. Aside from safety issues, these therapies are difficult and expensive to produce.

Nanoparticles are also being investigated for their use in enhancing diagnostic imaging, as contrast agents during an MRI, or to carry radioactive tracers during PET and CT scans. They can also be designed to bind to specific markers in cancer cells, improving accuracy and clarity in cancer diagnostics. Better diagnostics means earlier detection and earlier intervention.

Energy-based treatments physically interfere with cellular processes in the tumor. High-intensity focused ultrasound (HIFU) is an emerging technology that uses ultrasound waves to generate heat and ablate, or destroy, cancer cells. This localized process can be targeted with precision, thereby minimizing damage to healthy tissues. It is a treatment that can be repeated, and it is noninvasive, which means recovery time is shorter and there is a lower risk of complications.

The procedure is guided using imaging like MRI or ultrasound and, through the skin or using a probe, the doctor directs the high-frequency ultrasound waves, so their energy becomes focused at the tumor. There, they generate enough heat to destroy the cancer cells. It is a slow procedure and can take several hours to cover an entire tumor. HIFU is used to treat prostate cancer, and in some cases liver and kidney cancer in patients who are not candidates for surgery. It is also used to alleviate pain in pancreatic and bone cancer. HIFU remains an experimental treatment for many other cancers.

The drawbacks of this therapy are that it is primarily effective on small to medium tumors and in solid organs nearer the skin's surface. It is less effective where the waves have to travel through hollow spaces, as they get blocked or scattered. Also, there is energy loss over distance, so there are limits to how deeply it can penetrate. A pulse of the ultrasound only covers a tiny area, and as more overlapping pulses are needed, the treatment becomes less efficient and riskier. The side effects include burns and tissue damage, swelling, nerve damage, and fatigue.

Despite limitations, researchers are eager to explore further applications of this technology as it has fewer side effects than many standard treatments. It is currently being investigated as an alternative to surgery in breast cancer and is showing great potential as a noninvasive way to address brain tumors like glioblastoma.

Tumor treating fields (TTF) are another emerging energy-based therapy. TTFs use low-intensity alternating electrical fields to interfere with cancer cell division. These disruptions lead to cell death and slow the growth of the tumor. The treatment is delivered through transducer arrays attached to a wearable device, usually a cap. These adhesive electrode arrays are placed on the skin using MRI imaging, ensuring optimal positioning relative to the tumor's location. The arrays generate continuous low-intensity electrical fields, powered by a portable, battery-operated device. To be effective, the device must typically be worn eighteen to twenty hours per day. Tumor treating fields are a noninvasive localized therapy, which means they can be used alongside other treatments without interfering with them. This therapy is generally well tolerated and has no risk of toxicity.

Side effects include rashes, skin irritation, and dermatitis where the transducer arrays are attached. In some cases, the treatment can cause anemia and neutropenia, a condition caused by very low levels of immune cells called neutrophils. The long-term side effects and the impact of alternating electric fields on healthy tissue are still being investigated. The FDA has approved TTFs for the treatment of recurrent brain tumors called glioblastoma, and inoperable mesothelioma. Ongoing trials are investigating its potential for use against pancreatic, ovarian, lung, breast, renal and colorectal cancer.

The bulky equipment and battery pack, as well as the fact that it has to be used nearly continuously, are drawbacks. The high cost of the treatment is also a drawback. But it is low risk and has some proven benefit. Recent and ongoing studies are showing that TTFs are promising when used in combination with immunotherapy, chemotherapy, and radiation.

Hyperthermia uses high temperatures to destroy cancer cells and nearby blood vessels. Whole-body hyperthermia is being studied as a way to make chemotherapy and radiation more effective in treating metastatic cancer. The patient's body temperature is raised by using heating blankets or thermal chambers. Sometimes the temperatures are raised to simulate a fever, which is called fever-range whole-body hyperthermia. Studies suggest this may activate the immune system and raise the levels of cell-killing agents in the blood. Regional or isolation perfusion is a kind of hyperthermia in which an isolated blood supply is pumped into a heating device and returned to the body to heat the area.

Radiation therapies have also become increasingly targeted with the advent of precision medicine. Boron neutron capture therapy (BNCT) is an experimental targeted radiation therapy that uses boron-10 and neutron beams to destroy cancer cells. The patient is given a drug that carries boron-10 to the tumor, where it selectively accumulates in the cancer cells. These are then exposed to a low-energy neutron beam. When the neutrons interact with the boron-10, the reaction releases high-energy radiation inside the tumor. Because this radiation only travels a short distance, the process minimizes the damage to surrounding healthy tissue. Although the technique itself is not new, advances in modern neutron generators and more efficient carrier drugs are renewing interest in its use. It is attractive because it can be highly targeted and localized, which means the therapy can be completed in fewer sessions and with less toxicity than traditional radiation.

So far only Japan is allowing the clinical use of BNCT, other countries including the United States are still in clinical trials. Although it is a promising technology, it faces some challenges including high cost and accessibility. In the past, the neutron source was limited to nuclear reactors. While specialized accelerators are now a more convenient alternative, they remain largely unavailable outside select research hospitals. Another challenge facing the therapy is that it is only effective if the boron-10 is properly taken up by the cancer cells. Research is focused on more effective and selective delivery drugs with reduced toxicity. The treatment has the potential for being a breakthrough for the precision treatment of brain tumors like glioblastoma, head and neck, and liver cancer, and melanoma.

Combination therapies are making previously untreatable cancers manageable because multi-pronged approaches seem better able to slow the development of aggressive malignancies. Precision, or personalized medicine is driving advances in cutting-edge cancer treatment by identifying the unique molecular characteristics of an individual's cancer and targeting these features with combination therapies. While past treatments often followed a one-size-fits-all approach, precision medicine is paving the way for a more tailored and integrative approach to cancer care. Cancer cells that do not respond to a single treatment are more likely to adapt and become resistant. Going after more than one target at a time is a critical shift in current treatment models which could prevent or delay that kind of resistance. Current studies are showing that monotherapy, the use of a single type of treatment, is more likely to fail.

ComboMATCH (Combination Therapy Platform Trial with Molecular Analysis for Therapy Choice) is a group of ongoing clinical trials launched by the National Cancer Institute (NCI) to find out whether using drug combinations can overcome the treatment resistance that occurs when using a single drug targeting a single mutation. This precision medicine cancer initiative is the largest of its kind to evaluate combinations of treatments that block both the drivers of tumor growth and their mechanisms of resistance.

New biomedical technologies have completely transformed the landscape of cancer research, but there are benefits and drawbacks. For example, gene editing tools present serious ethical questions involving informed consent, genetic modification, and long-term repercussions. DNA sequencing technologies have made it possible to investigate cancer down to the smallest molecular detail, but they have also raised questions about the significance and usefulness of the data generated.

Technological innovations find their way to clinical practice very slowly, and just because these innovations receive a lot of press, it does not mean practicing physicians are trained or competent in their use. Having heard the hype, the public expects better medical insights and improved outcomes, but the hype is simply not yet standard of care. When expectations have not been met, technology can sometimes be seen as failing.

Cutting-edge therapies must not only demonstrate the potential to improve patient outcomes and be supported by strong research, but they must also meet standards of cost and accessibility. New therapies have a limited impact if patients cannot take advantage of them. Financial implications for both patients and the health care system are also key considerations before a treatment can go from cutting-edge to standard care.

40. Is complementary or alternative medicine an option?

Complementary and alternative medicine are terms that are sometimes used interchangeably to describe therapies, products, practices, and systems which are not part of mainstream medicine. Usually, if a treatment is complementary, it is used alongside standard medical care.

Complementary medicine refers to treatments that can manage symptoms and side effects and improve overall quality of life. They are not, in and of themselves, considered to be standard medical care, and although they are generally considered beneficial, there is less research available to support their effectiveness.

Alternative medicine, on the other hand, replaces conventional treatments like chemotherapy or radiation. It often refers to untested or even disproven methods, or methods that simply lack any robust scientific evidence of safety and effectiveness.

In the United States, conventional medicine (which is also called mainstream medicine, biomedicine, allopathic, Western, or orthodox medicine) is the standard system of care. Medical professionals treat symptoms and diseases using widely accepted methods backed by scientific research and clinical studies. In speaking of complementary and alternative medicine, people are usually referring to natural, naturopathic, or holistic medicine, or healing systems and beliefs from another country or culture. Some of these treatments are backed by scientific research, but on the whole, there is less evidence of safety and effectiveness.

People with cancer consider using complementary and alternative medicine for a variety of reasons. Often, they simply want to do everything possible to get better and will explore all options. Treatment approaches that may have fewer side effects are attractive when compared to the harsh reality of many standard cancer treatments, and therapies that are considered "natural" are perceived as being safer. And because a cancer diagnosis can be a devastating shock, many patients find comfort in being able to take some control over their health.

Success stories, testimonials, individual claims, and anecdotal accounts are often compelling and provide hope, even if they are without a basis in science. Social influence can also play a role as patients are exposed to a much larger network of input than ever before. Some patients simply become frustrated or dissatisfied with conventional therapy. They have, or can develop, a mistrust of mainstream medicine. In some cases, opting for alternative treatment is an economic choice because it is perceived as being cheaper or more accessible.

Patients from certain cultural backgrounds may also gravitate to an approach to health that aligns with their personal, religious, or cultural views, such as Ayurvedic medicine or traditional Chinese medicine, which are healing systems and beliefs that have long histories and traditions in other parts of the world.

Many people in the United States today are increasingly drawn to the idea of holistic health, which addresses the whole person, body, mind, and spirit. They find many of the integrative aspects of complementary and alternative treatments more appealing. Naturopathic strategies often address things like lifestyle factors, overall wellness, and immune function, whereas conventional medicine focuses mainly on the disease.

A 2023 survey published in *JCO Oncology Practice* revealed that 70 percent of cancer patients said they used complementary medicine in addition to their conventional cancer treatment. Health care providers can serve their patients better when they understand their patients' motivations, but ultimately, the decision to use complementary and alternative therapies rests with the patient. Patients who have strong feelings about specific treatments can, and should, outline them in an advance care plan so their wishes will be honored. (See Question 44—What is palliative care and why is it important to consider end-of-life issues?)

Complementary treatments that help cancer patients cope with the symptoms and side effects of conventional cancer treatments are also generally accepted and recommended by oncologists in the United States. Studies show that cancer support groups and cognitive and emotional intervention like psychotherapy and counseling lead to better quality of life during cancer treatment. Some evidence suggests that mind and body practices, like meditation, biofeedback, spirituality and prayer, hypnosis, music and relaxation therapy, and imagery are helpful in reducing stress and managing pain. These therapies can provide emotional and psychological support over the course of cancer treatment.

Yoga has been recognized as an activity that can improve physical fitness, reduce fatigue, and support emotional well-being. Studies show it reduces anxiety and improves quality of life. Tai chi and dance therapy, which focus on slow movement and controlled breathing, have also been shown to relax the body and mind. Medical professionals will usually encourage any physical activity that is tolerated by the patient. These strategies can provide physical and psychological relief, and although some of them need more research to prove consistent effectiveness, they are generally considered beneficial.

Manipulative and body-based practices like massage, chiropractic therapy, and reflexology have limited evidence of benefit, but oncologists may recommend them to manage symptoms or pain, especially nerve pain caused by chemotherapy. Research does show, however, that acupuncture can be effective in managing symptoms of cancer and its treatment, such as pain and nausea. For safety, patients receiving this kind of supportive care should only get it from therapists who are qualified to treat people with cancer.

Energy healing like reiki or therapeutic touch focuses on balancing the energy flow in the body. There is no scientific evidence to support its effectiveness, but it has no harmful effects, and some patients seem to find it beneficial.

Nutrition-based complementary practices like naturopathy and homeopathy can include vitamins, dietary supplements, botanicals like herbs, and other special foods or diets. There is no evidence that these alone can control cancer, but optimizing nutrition during cancer treatment is important.

Although some limited research shows intermittent fasting and caloric restriction could be beneficial, doctors will usually encourage patients to eat anything they can tolerate because they want to avoid dangerous weight loss. Relying on a specific diet without professional guidance could also lead to nutritional deficiencies. Some patients may prefer to work with a nutritionist that is qualified to advise cancer patients, because dietary changes should be handled carefully.

Oncologists will generally advise against most supplements and herbs during ongoing therapy because many of them react or interact with cancer treatments and drugs, potentially making them either less effective or more toxic. Patients wanting to pursue nutrition-based therapies should always consult with a specialist to be safe.

Some studies suggest maintaining healthy vitamin D levels may improve cancer treatment outcomes. Research into high-dose intravenous vitamin C has shown promise, but how much it might interfere with other treatments is still unclear. There is mixed evidence that ginger might help control chemotherapy-induced nausea. The Food and Drug Administration (FDA) has approved the medical use of cannabis for cancer patients with issues like pain, nausea, stress, sleep, and anxiety. And while an increasing number of people are using it to help manage their symptoms and side effects, cannabis can also cause its own health complications. Other drawbacks include cost, safety, and potential legal issues.

A common misconception about botanicals and supplements is that if something is natural it is safe. Another misconception is that if a little is good, more will be better. Many compounds in plants are toxic, which is one reason they provide the basis of so many potent drugs. Mega-doses of vitamins can also be potentially harmful. And just because a folk remedy has been around for a long time does not always mean its long-term safety or potential interactions have been properly tested. Natural does not necessarily mean safe and effective.

The FDA regulates dietary supplements differently than foods and drugs. Manufacturers must follow the FDA's Good Manufacturing Practice Standards which require that nutritional supplements be safe and that the labels be accurate about ingredients, nutritional content, and warnings. They do not require the manufacturers to prove the effectiveness of the supplements, however.

Consumer Reports, a non-profit consumer advocacy organization, recommends looking for third-party certification on the label like USP, consumerlabs.com, NSF international, and UL solutions when choosing a supplement. These independent laboratories verify the quality, purity, and potency of the product, and give assurances that the product is what it claims to be and is free from harmful contaminants.

To develop the most effective treatment plan, the health care team needs a comprehensive understanding of what the patient is currently doing and taking before treatment begins, as well as any changes they may consider during treatment. It is essential to consult with a health care provider about anything that could interact with cancer therapy. It is also important to choose a complementary therapy provider carefully. Ideally, they should have experience treating cancer patients and be able to cater to their unique requirements. Useful sources of information about using complementary therapies during cancer treatment are the National Institutes of Health's National Center for Complementary and Integrative Health (NCCIH), and the National Cancer Institute's Office of Cancer Complementary and Alternative Medicine (OCCAM).

Some cancer patients choose to avoid conventional cancer treatment altogether and decide to use alternative therapy exclusively. Common choices include high-dose vitamin treatments or herbal therapies like tinctures and teas, special or extreme diets, homeopathic or naturopathic medicine, spiritual healing, and energy healing. Although these methods may provide some benefits in certain cases, most of them lack any evidence of effectiveness and none has been scientifically shown to cure cancer.

The biggest risk in using alternative therapies to replace mainstream treatments is disease progression. The longer a more effective treatment is delayed, the worse the prognosis becomes, because a more advanced cancer is harder to treat. And because alternative treatments are not supported by as much research, side effects, interactions, and complications are more difficult to anticipate. Many of them have never been tested on pregnant or breastfeeding women, if they have been tested at all. These kinds of treatments also tend to offer less oversight and monitoring.

Patients who choose alternative therapies instead of conventional ones have a substantially lower chance of survival. According to a 2017 study published in the *Journal of the National Cancer Institute*, cancer patients who chose alternative medicine therapies as the sole treatment for their cancers were more than twice as likely to die compared with patients who chose conventional cancer treatments.

Insurance may sometimes cover some well-known complementary and alternative methods like homeopathy or naturopathy, but it is unlikely to cover anything that does not have proven benefits for a particular diagnosis. In addition, complementary and alternative medicine providers are less likely to take any insurance, let alone your particular insurance, so these treatments, even if they are considered generally safe and approved by your oncology team, may be costly.

This is why, when faced with patients who refuse conventional treatment in favor of alternative therapies, oncologists will try to educate them as much as possible. If the alternative treatment is ineffective, patients need to know if conventional therapy will still be an option. Patients who pursue this course often find it difficult to communicate with their health care team and sometimes do not disclose their decision. This can strain the doctor-patient relationship and result in a breakdown in trust and collaboration.

The implications of refusing evidence-based medicine can be quite serious. And yet personal stories and anecdotal evidence can be quite compelling. Although the statistics are not in favor of alternative treatments, there always seem to be miraculous exceptions and a patient in this position is bound to hold out hope that they might be one of them.

Miracle cure stories are common, but documented cases of cancer being cured without treatment are rare and difficult to explain. Some cases may simply be the result of a misdiagnosis or overdiagnosis, meaning the cancer was slow growing, unlikely to cause harm, and might never have required treatment in the first place. In other cases, a change in diet or other lifestyle modification may have boosted the immune system, improving the body's ability to fight the disease. If this change coincided with the alternative therapy, it might be mistaken for effectiveness, but these changes alone are very unlikely to have long-term effect or cure aggressive cancer.

Proponents of unproven alternative treatments sometimes cite spontaneous remission as evidence that the treatment has "cured" the cancer. Spontaneous regression or remission refers to the unexpected or unexplained reduction or complete disappearance of cancer without the use of conventional treatment. This event is rare, occurring in fewer than one in 60,000 to 100,000 cancer cases, but it has been well documented, especially in relation to certain cancers like leukemia, melanoma, and neuroblastoma. The reason this happens is unknown, but may be related to immune system activation, possibly because of infection or interference with the tumor microenvironment. Hormonal changes or genetic factors may also impact this kind of healing. But it is important to understand that the only link between alternative therapy and spontaneous remission is anecdotal, and that rigorous scientific evidence is lacking.

There is also such a thing as survivorship bias, the focus being on the small sample of people who experienced a positive outcome and ignoring the large sample of people who did not. We hear from those who survive but not from those for whom treatment was ineffective. Sometimes patients will undergo a conventional treatment and assume it was ineffective, and a positive outcome is attributed to subsequent therapy. It is always important to distinguish correlation from causation, just because one event happened after another, does not mean the first event caused the second.

The placebo effect is a real phenomenon in which a patient experiences improvement in symptoms after receiving fake or non-active treatment, due entirely to their expectations and beliefs. And although it is unlikely to eliminate the cancer itself, it can be powerful and help people stay healthier longer than anyone thought possible.

A hard reality to keep in mind when watching or reading the success stories of alternative treatments is that even if they are not involved in actual fraud, certain people crave attention, especially online and on social media, and they may not be truthful about their treatments. They may simply claim miraculous survival when in fact their cure was the result of conventional treatment.

And of course, when desperate people are looking for answers in an environment that may involve a great deal of money and very little scientific evidence, the possibility of fraud is quite high. According to the American Cancer Society (ACS), one in three articles about cancer treatment on social media include incorrect or even harmful information, so careful research is indicated.

Being informed is vital when investigating these kinds of therapies. The FDA has warned the public to beware of fraudulent cancer treatments that are promoted online or on social media platforms. Always check the reliability of sources and question anyone making blanket statements about "cures." The ACS suggests looking for information on websites like the Office of Cancer Complementary and Alternative Medicine (OCCAM), and Quackwatch.org, a website that collects information on health frauds, myths, fads, fallacies, and misconduct. (See Question 41—What is the best way to look for cancer information on the internet?)

In some very rare cases, though, science is indeed baffled. There is much we still do not know about the disease. But the evidence still supports the fact that most cancers require proven medical intervention for the best chance of survival. When cancer patients consent to a course of treatment, they are potentially making a life-altering decision. They need to feel the treatment gives them the best possible chance based on available information. A fair question to ask when considering any cancer treatment, conventional or alternative, would be: "Given the evidence, how confident am I in this treatment?" This keeps the discussion rational, fact-based, and patient-centered.

Doctors and patients alike would agree that a personalized, evidence-based approach is the most important consideration in treating cancer. This is in part why the popularity of integrative medicine has increased lately in the United States. Integrative medicine combines conventional medicine with evidence-based complementary practices to support overall well-being. This approach, along with holistic medicine which focuses on physical, mental, and spiritual health, encompasses all the individual patient's preferences and needs.

The interest in integrative medicine has spurred increased research into many complementary therapies, which would increase the level of confidence for patients and medical professionals alike. Taking charge and advocating for your health with a health care team that can advise and help make safe and informed choices should help cancer patients avail themselves of all the benefits offered by non-traditional medicine.

41. What is the best way to look for cancer information on the internet?

Although the internet might be the first place you look for information about cancer, it may not always be easy to distinguish what is true and safe, what is an advertisement, or what is straight up falsehood. Cancer information on the internet may come from a variety of sources, and it may be objective and educational, biased, or commercial, or it could be a scam, spam, or con. Because it is anonymous and far-reaching, and because it is easier to appear legitimate online than in the real world, the internet can be extremely misleading.

Information found online should come from trusted and credible sources like government agencies, hospitals, universities, and medical journals and books. But ultimately, information is just that. It is meant to inform and educate. It should never take the place of medical advice.

Scientific data can also be difficult to interpret, so even stories published by news agencies may be misrepresented, sensationalized, or inaccurate. Some headlines use scare tactics as clickbait, some sites may support very specific viewpoints or agendas. It might be hard to tell if the information is accurate or balanced. Cancer research is also a rapidly evolving field, but outdated or debunked information can still be found online.

Searches can turn up commercial or sponsored results as well. The information on these websites might be interesting or useful, but their agenda is to promote products or services. Online health personalities often have compelling and thorough podcasts and videos, but ultimately, they may also be selling books or programs.

Increasingly, people are turning to artificial intelligence (AI) like ChatGPT for health information, which certainly has some advantages. It is accessible, private, and quick. It breaks down complex information into fairly simple language and provides good broad overviews of many topics. But AI is a tool, and not qualified to offer medical advice. It is only as accurate as the information it can access, so it could be outdated or incomplete. The biggest risk is that people will trust information delivered this way and delay seeking medical advice. (See Question 46—What is the future direction of cancer research?)

The internet, and social media in particular, is full of people who have no medical expertise offering tips and information. Watching people tell their personal cancer stories can be reassuring and informative, but a viral TikTok video should not be trusted to deliver valid, proven, cancer treatment and prevention strategies. Online support groups and chat rooms allow people to connect and still remain anonymous if they wish, but they are not the best sources for accurate or current information.

And not all misinformation about cancer comes from the simply misinformed. There are hackers and online fraudsters who exploit desperate people, and a cancer diagnosis can make people vulnerable and desperate. Someone in that situation may cling to what they want to see or hear without question or suspicion, making them easy to prey upon. Claims like "treats all forms of cancer," "cures cancer," or "selectively kills cancer cells" should be automatic red flags.

So how can you be sure you are looking at trustworthy websites? The National Cancer Institute (NCI) suggests asking certain questions, such as "Who manages the information or website?" "Is the website asking for personal information?" "How up to date is the information?" The domain suffix, or letters at the end of the web address, can make it clear whether it is a government website (.gov), or a website run by an educational institution (.edu). These are good sources. Websites ending in .org (usually a non-profit organization) or .com (usually commercial or private) may also be trusted sites but should be looked at more carefully. For example, a non-profit funded by a private company and heavily featuring ads might raise some questions. Medical and cancer treatment centers like the Mayo Clinic, or MD Anderson Cancer Center can be good sources, with up-to-date information and patient resources, but they may emphasize their own specialties and services and might not provide comprehensive answers.

Sometimes web addresses feature a two-letter country code after the URL. Treatment availability or statistics might not be relevant to someone doing research in the United States if the website is from Australia (.au) or Belgium (.be). In the "About Us" section, it should be clear whether the site is selling or promoting a "cure." How the information on the site is documented should also be easy to tell. There should be scientific references and links. Check for dates and updates, because even cancer information that is a couple of years old might be inaccurate or incomplete today.

Some red flags might include outlandish or miraculous claims, testimonials but no scientific data, payment in advance, or money back guarantees. Cancer scams can be reported to the Federal Trade Commission (FTC). The Food and Drug Administration (FDA), which is responsible for regulating drugs and setting standards for supplements, is a great resource for checking up on any unproven claims.

Trusted places to begin looking for information about cancer include the National Cancer Institute(NCI) (www.cancer.gov), and the American Cancer Society (ACS) (www.cancer.org), which has its own secure online community for cancer survivors and their families called the Cancer Survivors Network. The National Library of Medicine and MedlinePlus are useful resources for finding scientific articles, medical studies, and symptom checkers. Other helpful government sites include the Centers for Disease Control and Prevention (CDC), the Environmental Protection Agency (EPA), the National Institutes of

Health (NIH), the World Health Organization (WHO), and the Food and Drug Administration (FDA).

42. What are the long-term health concerns after cancer treatment?

After their final treatment, each cancer patient rings the bell signifying a major milestone in their cancer journey. It is a wonderful way to acknowledge all of the things that have been overcome up to this point and marks the beginning of a new chapter. Whether the patient is in complete remission, meaning the signs and symptoms of the cancer are gone, or they are keeping the disease at bay with some form of maintenance therapy, long-term health remains an important consideration for cancer survivors even as the focus shifts from active treatment to ongoing care. Long-term health concerns vary and depend on the type of cancer and treatment, but many survivors face significant challenges that affect their overall health and quality of life.

Even if a cancer patient is in remission, they may still have to live with many long-term physical side effects of the disease and its treatment. Toxicity from chemotherapy, cellular damage from radiation, and the ravages of surgery can all result in pain. In fact, over a third of cancer survivors report living with chronic pain. Even more report fatigue that lasts long after treatment is over. This is often due to the immune system being left weakened by the disease and the treatments. This can also result in increased vulnerability to infections and lasting effects on bone marrow function.

Cognitive impairment is another common long-term effect. It is often referred to as "chemo brain" as patients find it difficult to concentrate and process information. Chemotherapy-induced peripheral neuropathy in the hands and feet is another neurological side effect. This is a result of treatment toxicity that can take years to dissipate, if ever. Some treatments, particularly chemotherapy and radiation, leave lasting damage in the organs, leading to cardiovascular issues, liver or kidney damage, and lung problems like fibrosis. Patients often have lingering digestive and nutritional issues, especially as a result of cancer in the digestive tract. These issues can result in muscle wasting, weight loss, and bowel dysfunction.

Treatments including some surgical procedures, hormone therapy, and chemotherapy can lead to hormonal changes resulting in low bone density, joint pain, and stiffness, and even reproductive health issues like early menopause and infertility. A type of swelling and fluid retention known as lymphedema is a common and significant long-term effect, especially for survivors of breast cancer and other cancers where the lymph nodes have been removed or irradiated. And finally, many cancer treatments increase the risk of getting a new, unrelated, or secondary cancer.

Research into the psychological effects of cancer and its treatment has shown that a patient might be cured of the disease but may still suffer long-lasting mental issues akin to trauma. The largest psychological impact of cancer is the anxiety caused by the fear of the cancer coming back. Recurrence, when the cancer returns months or years after treatment ends, is a possibility for all cancer survivors. Many survivors experience anxiety, depression, and other mental health problems. Findings estimate that symptoms of post-traumatic stress disorder (PTSD) are reported in around 5 to 19 percent of cancer patients.

One of the psychological impacts of cancer is that it can lead to withdrawal from social interactions. That feeling of isolation can last long past the end of cancer treatments. And many therapies, especially surgery, can affect physical appearance and body function. Studies show the impact to self-esteem and body image is especially significant among younger survivors.

It is important to address these issues in order to optimize recovery and long-term well-being. Cancer survivors need consistent and careful monitoring, and a care approach that might also include psychotherapists, dietitians, physical therapists, and palliative care professionals. Physical activity and tailored exercise programs have been shown to improve symptoms like pain, fatigue, and peripheral neuropathy. Acupuncture and other complementary therapies may also help in managing long-term side effects. Cognitive behavioral therapy is used to mitigate the effects of "chemo brain," and ongoing psychological support can help teach useful coping mechanisms. Supportive networks, family, and friends are just as important after treatment has ended as they were before. Psychological side effects should be considered when developing personalized care plans to enhance cancer survivorship.

This does not mean that cancer survivors should become hyper focused on their health. This would simply turn into another source of anxiety. The idea is that taking control and becoming more proactive about their health, making better lifestyle choices, and rediscovering their resilience, is a positive step forward.

As harsh as the disease and its treatments can be, many cancer survivors find the experience has brought them new perspectives and strengths. Some say it was a wake-up call, that they have developed a deeper appreciation for life and learned to prioritize what truly matters. Others discover a new sense of purpose, a motivation for personal growth, inspiring them to pursue dreams or make major life changes. Many find they have made deep personal connections with family, friends, and support networks, and the shift in perspective has led them to greater gratitude and mindfulness.

43. What happens if the treatment fails, or if the cancer comes back?

Cancer recurrence means the cancer has returned after a period of remission. It is the result of some cancer cells remaining undetectable in the body after treatment. Some oncologists compare metastatic cancer to spilling seeds onto a shag carpet. You can vacuum it repeatedly and not see any seeds, but there are probably still some in there, and there is no way to know for sure. This means that although the treatment may result in no more visible signs of cancer, the cancer cells may not have been completely eradicated.

Sometimes, cancer recurrence is caused by treatment resistance. Cancer treatments can put selective pressure on cancer cells. The cells may simply no longer be susceptible to a particular therapy because they were inherently resistant, or they evolved to resist. And resistant cells flourish once the other cells are destroyed. This means the treatment has failed. The first thing the cancer care team will look at is other treatment options they have not yet explored. They will also investigate the possibility that a new drug has been approved that may better target the cancer. (See Question 15—Are you more likely to get cancer if you have had it before?)

In some cases, physicians may suggest using a drug that is not necessarily a cancer drug. Off-label drug use, which is the use of a Food and Drug Administration (FDA)-approved drug for a condition that is not specified on the packaging, is common in cancer treatment. The drug may be approved for another disease, a different kind of cancer, or in a different dosage, but emerging research may suggest alternative uses. The drug may target molecular pathways shared by other cancers or show promise in being used in combination with other therapies. Using a drug off-label requires a physician's approval and careful consideration of risks and benefits. There is usually a good scientific rationale for using a drug in this way, and physicians will recommend it because it is potentially beneficial, it can address an unmet need, or it can help tailor a new treatment.

The drawback of off-label drug use is that there is less clinical data and therefore less information about its effectiveness and potential side effects under these new conditions. Cost can be an issue because insurance companies only cover off-label drug use under very specific circumstances.

Using drugs off-label is not unusual in cancer treatment. In fact, some FDA-approved cancer immunotherapy drugs are based on repurposing existing drugs, like thalidomide and tamoxifen, and many more are being tested as potential cancer therapies. The advantage in repurposing or expanding the uses of existing drugs is that the research and safety data already exist. This accelerated development means the drug can become accessible sooner and at lower cost.

Exploring clinical trials can be another way cancer patients can look for treatment options beyond standard therapies. Clinical trials are a way to access new drugs, therapies, procedures, and devices, as well as supportive and palliative care, that are not yet widely available. They are also an opportunity to contribute to research.

Patients can find out about relevant clinical trials by speaking with their care team or searching online databases for ongoing trials. Good resources include ClinicalTrials.gov, the National Cancer Institute (NCI) Clinical Trial Finder, cancer center websites like Memorial Sloan Kettering or Mayo Clinic, and patient advocacy groups like the American Cancer Society (ACS).

Patients wishing to participate in clinical trials need to weigh the potential risks and side effects. They will go through a process of informed consent so they fully understand the trial before they enroll. This process involves disclosing to potential subjects the information needed to make an informed decision, helping them understand what this information means, and ensuring they are deciding freely, without undue influence.

Participating in a clinical trial can provide a patient with emerging experimental treatments that might not yet be widely available. These may be more effective than standard treatments, especially for aggressive or treatment-resistant cancers. During a clinical trial, participants are closely monitored by specialists and researchers, receiving comprehensive medical care, with frequent imaging and tests to track their progress. And no matter the outcome, participants often feel good about contributing to cancer research and helping future patients. Ultimately, there is always a chance their participation will lead to a breakthrough treatment that can improve survival or quality of life. (See Question 39—What are current cutting-edge cancer treatments?)

But there is no guarantee that the experimental drug will work as expected or be more effective than standard care. Many trials have specific requirements for eligibility, and not all patients will qualify. Some patients may receive a placebo or standard treatment instead of the new drug, although cancer trials rarely use placebos alone. An experimental drug may have unexpected or very severe side effects, and its long-term effects may not be fully known. Participation is a commitment that may require frequent trips and hospital visits. If the treatment proves to be ineffective or unsafe the study could be stopped early. Costs can include the experimental treatment itself, tests, doctor visits, travel, and lodging. These are sometimes covered by the study or support organizations. Insurance coverage for experimental treatments varies.

Clinical trials are not just an option for patients whose treatment has failed, patients at any stage of cancer may participate, as long as they are eligible. Many studies also look at screening and prevention, and some are even open to people who do not have a cancer diagnosis but may be at elevated risk.

Cancer patients can sometimes access experimental treatments outside of clinical trials. The Expanded Access Program, formerly called Compassionate Use, is an FDA-regulated program that was established in the 1980s to help HIV/AIDS patients access investigational drugs. Patients who qualify for this program have serious or life-threatening conditions, have exhausted standard treatments, are ineligible for a clinical trial, and have no other therapy available to them. A physician submits the request to the FDA. The FDA and an Institutional Review Board examine the request to ensure patient safety and ethical consideration, and if it is approved, and the manufacturer agrees to provide the drug, the patient goes through an informed consent process to make sure they understand the potential risks.

The Right to Try Act, which was passed in 2018, is a law that allows terminally ill patients to access investigational drugs without requiring FDA approval. It is meant to speed up the process to help patients with a life-threatening disease who have exhausted all standard treatment options and are ineligible for a clinical trial. The experimental drug must have already completed a phase 1 clinical trial and still be seeking FDA approval. The physician submits a request directly to the drug manufacturer. No FDA involvement is required. If the manufacturer agrees to provide the drug, the patient goes through the informed consent process.

Although the Right to Try Act provides a faster route with less regulation, there are higher risks because there is no FDA oversight. The Expanded Access Program can delay treatment because of its review process requirement, but it offers more safety monitoring and collects real-world data from patients using the experimental drugs.

In either case, the drug manufacturers are not legally required to provide the drug. And although most insurance plans cover some of the costs relating to taking part in a clinical trial, they may not cover experimental treatment alone.

44. What is palliative care and why is it important to consider end-of-life issues?

Palliative care is specialized medical care that focuses on improving quality of life by managing pain, reducing side effects and symptoms, and providing emotional and psychological support. It tends to have a more integrated approach, and its goal is to address the patient as a whole, not so much to cure but to provide comfort and relief from the disease and from the treatment.

There has been a recent shift toward integrating palliative care earlier in the cancer treatment process. This kind of care is no longer restricted to end-of-life care, it can be started at any point from the time of the initial diagnosis and given alongside curative or life-extending care. Studies show that patients receiving palliative care experience fewer hospitalizations and are less likely to receive aggressive care near the end of life. They also report a higher quality of life and experience longer survival times. Palliative care consultations result in better communication about the patient's wishes and more effective management of symptoms and pain. The American Society of Clinical Oncology recommends that all patients with advanced cancer receive palliative care.

Patients can be referred to palliative care specialists by their oncology care team, and several national organizations, like the Center to Advance Palliative Care or the National Hospice and Palliative Care Organization, have databases for referrals. Insurance coverage varies by state, but some kind of palliative service is usually covered, especially when it involves symptom management.

Pain management and symptom control are the main physical issues addressed by palliative care. It often involves using cancer therapies like chemotherapy and radiation to alleviate pain and discomfort, even if they cannot cure. Other physical symptoms that are helped with drugs and complementary therapies include fatigue, nausea, shortness of breath, and insomnia.

Specialists in palliative care can also provide emotional, psychological, and spiritual support. They can assist in finding resources to help with depression, anxiety, and fear, which are common but less acknowledged challenges for cancer patients. They can also access nutritional support and suggest integrative therapies like acupuncture, yoga, and meditation to help with stress, pain, and discomfort. (See Question 40—Is complementary or alternative medicine an option?)

And the role of palliative care also extends beyond helping the patient. Because family and friends are an important part of a patient's support system, and because these caregivers can also feel overwhelmed or helpless, palliative care specialists are trained to help them cope and find support.

The most important aspect of palliative care is the coordination of care. This means ensuring there is a flow of communication between the patient, the oncologists, and any other specialist on the medical care team. They can also assist with financial, insurance, and legal issues, and, crucially, guide the patient through advance care planning.

Advance care planning is the process of discussing and documenting the patient's choices concerning medical and end-of-life care to make sure their wishes are respected if they become unable to communicate. This type of legal planning can help patients articulate their preferences about the extent of medical intervention they are willing to accept. It is about optimizing their comfort and preserving their dignity. Having these conversations helps patients and their families navigate financial, legal, medical, and emotional burdens with clarity and support.

An important part of the plan is creating an advance directive to outline the patient's wishes. This includes a living will, which is a document that states whether or not the patient wishes to receive certain types of life-sustaining measures, such as the use of machines to be kept alive like ventilators, tube feeding, withholding food and fluids, and organ and tissue donation. It might also include "do not resuscitate" orders (DNR) which are instructions to not use CPR if breathing stops. Patients have the right to electively forego lifesaving or life-sustaining medical intervention. The advance directive might also include whether and when the patient wants to abandon treatment, or try for experimental treatment.

Another legal document to include in an advance directive is a durable power of attorney for health care. Also known as a health care proxy, or medical power of attorney, it designates a trusted person to make medical decisions on the patient's behalf. Appointing someone in advance helps ensure the patient's wishes are honored, even in situations that are not explicitly addressed in a living will. It allows for critical decisions to be made in an emergency and is legally recognized by health care providers. This way, the patient can extend their control beyond their ability to make decisions. It is important to go through this process early, while the patient is still relatively healthy and while they are capable of giving informed consent. It ensures the choices are based on accurate information, prevents misunderstandings, and provides legal and ethical clarity.

Many patients feel that although they cannot protect their loved ones from what they may feel when the time comes, they can at least prepare them. These are difficult and overwhelming decisions to make, which might seem insurmountable once the patient is debilitated by the disease. Having these considerations set down in writing not only avoids future family conflicts but provides peace of mind for loved ones who will also not be thinking too clearly once the disease becomes advanced. And changes to advance directives can be made at any time, the process should be ongoing.

Most health care facilities have specialists who can assist patients through these steps. Once complete, copies of the advance care plan should go to members of the medical team, to family, and be kept in a safe and accessible place. It is important to keep in mind that the legal format or requirements of advance directives may change from state to state. Each state's legal aid office or bar association can provide more information.

In the case of advanced or terminal cancer, the priorities will shift. The care team may discuss the benefits and burdens of continued treatment versus comfort-focused care. This is when the patient may choose to consider hospice care. Whereas palliative care can be used during any stage of cancer care, hospice care begins when treatment that is meant to cure or control the disease is no longer effective or desired. Both focus on pain relief, emotional support, and quality of life, but hospice is a specialized form of palliative care that emphasizes the final stage of life. It helps patients live as comfortably and meaningfully as possible, ensuring their dignity and reducing their suffering. Hospice care can be given at home, which allows the patient to remain in a familiar setting rather than in a hospital. Otherwise, it can be given in a nursing home, or at a hospice facility.

And although hospice care focuses on comfort and dignity in the final days, a small number of patients facing a terminal diagnosis are looking for greater control over the time and circumstances of their death. This may lead some to difficult but important discussions about receiving medical aid in dying, which is also known as physician-assisted suicide. The legal right to end one's life is an ethically and legally complex issue which tries to balance patient autonomy with moral objections and fear of abuse. Medical aid in dying is legal in California, Colorado, Hawaii, Maine, Montana, New Jersey, New Mexico, Oregon, Vermont, Washington, and the District of Columbia, as long as the patient meets the medical and psychiatric requirements. According to data from these states, less than 1 percent of all deaths are attributed to physician-assisted death, but terminal cancer is the most common underlying disease in these cases.

A proactive approach toward addressing end-of-life issues is essential to receiving the highest quality of care and support. It reduces uncertainty and distress for patients and families, ensures that medical care aligns with the patient's values and goals, allows for better symptom control and higher quality of life.

45. How can I support someone who has cancer?

Supporting someone with cancer means being there for them, emotionally and physically. A cancer diagnosis can be very isolating, and studies show that no, or low, emotional support can be a stronger predictor of low quality of life than the cancer diagnosis itself. The kind of support you choose to offer may depend on the individual and your relationship with them.

Emotional support means being present and listening without judgment. Acknowledging the struggle while offering hope. At the beginning it may be hard to act normal around someone with a cancer diagnosis, but most people with cancer crave normalcy. It provides comfort and stability. This is why caregivers, family, and friends should be positive and realistic, and try not to treat cancer patients as if they were helpless. It is best to avoid making their diagnosis their whole identity.

Some people find it hard to accept support and feel they still need independence, so it is wise to be patient and respectful of their feelings and choices. They might not feel comfortable asking for support, or feel very isolated, so any sign that you are thinking of them, small acts of kindness or thoughtfulness, can help them feel supported. Cancer patients should know that many family members and friends feel it is an honor and privilege to take care of their loved one, and they should not worry about being a burden.

Sometimes it is difficult to know what to say, but it is better to share genuine feelings rather than be uncomfortably silent or artificially cheerful. Avoid saying things like "I know how you feel," because even if you have had a similar experience, you may not have felt the same way they do. It is more honest to say, "I don't know what to say," or "I am sorry this has happened." Let them know you are available to do things or just talk, and consider visiting often, not just on holidays and weekends. Try not to compare their experience with other people's and avoid discussing past behaviors that might be related to their illness.

Some cancer patients dislike being told they are "battling" cancer because it implies that they might not be fighting hard enough and if they tried a little more the outcome would be different. Urging them to be strong and brave, no matter how well-intentioned, may put pressure on them to act a certain way when, in fact, they feel very differently. They may feel anger and resentment toward their health care team, or healthy people, or God.

Offering practical support involves doing things to help alleviate the pressures of going through cancer treatment. This could mean helping with errands or accompanying them to medical appointments and treatment sessions and sitting with them. Suggesting activities or complementary therapies to support their well-being during treatment might be welcome. It also feels good to offer small gifts that center on pampering and self-care.

It is unwise to offer medical advice or opinions on things like diet and vitamins. They will already be inundated with health information and should be relying on the expert input of their medical team. It would be more helpful to assist them in finding a second opinion if they want one, or to help them research things they are trying to learn about by making sure the sources are fact-based and reliable. (See Question 41—What is the best way to find cancer information on the internet?)

Studies show that strong social networks and emotional support systems are consistently linked to better overall health outcomes. Social support is critical because maintaining strong ties can help reduce feelings of isolation and improve mental health. Peer support groups can enhance emotional resilience and provide insights. Engagement and connecting with others not only give a cancer patient comfort and motivation, but also play a role in improved immune function and healing.

Health advocacy may be an important way to help someone with cancer, as they may suddenly be overwhelmed by medical information and unable to recall everything they are told. Patients find it useful to have someone with them who can help communicate with medical professionals, ask questions, and take notes. In addition, they may appreciate help in managing their insurance matters, including understanding coverage and verifying benefits.

Financial and legal issues can also be difficult to navigate for someone in poor health. Financial worries are common and stressful with a cancer diagnosis. Patients may need support in dealing with insurance and medical billing, or legal planning such as advance directives and powers of attorney. Sometimes it is enough to simply have someone who can help research and clarify these subjects, fill in paperwork, or just access resources. Financial support might also mean offering financial assistance, accessing financial aid, or organizing a fundraiser.

A cancer diagnosis can induce a wide range of emotions, including shock, fear, anxiety, anger, and helplessness, and many people are overwhelmed or numb at first. This can make knowing what to say and do difficult. Each person's response is unique and can change throughout their experience. Whether they are negative and withdrawn, or working toward acceptance, you should support how they feel and respect their decisions, even if you disagree. The most important thing is to meet that person where they are and give them grace.

46. What is the future direction of cancer research?

There are many broad trends and technologies shaping the future of cancer research and how it will evolve over the next decade. New fields and technologies are driving the development of cancer detection, diagnostics, and treatment. At the forefront is precision medicine, which will be expanded with tools like liquid biopsies. New cancer biomarkers and new molecular pathways, as well as the role of cancer stem cells, will help refine treatment targets. The emerging field of spatial biology is rapidly expanding our understanding of cancer. And complementing these biological insights, artificial intelligence (AI) and computational oncology will enhance our ability to analyze complex data and predict outcomes. Finally, the study of the microbiome is beginning to reveal its potential role in influencing cancer development and treatment response.

Precision, or personalized, medicine will continue to be a driving force in the future of cancer research. The goal is to tailor disease prevention, detection, and treatment to the individual on a molecular level. Expanding this field will rely on precisely and affordably identifying individual genomic variations, both in the patient and in their cancer. The field of next-generation sequencing is revolutionizing precision medicine. Unlike the widely used Sanger sequencing, which sequences one fragment of DNA at a time, next generation sequencing simultaneously sequences millions of DNA fragments, making the process faster and more efficient. Genomics, which is the study of the entire human genome, including genes and their interactions, will also play a crucial role in cancer prevention. As genetic predispositions are identified, personalized risk assessments and interventions can be used, not only for early detection but potentially for prevention as well.

Liquid biopsies have emerged as an increasingly effective and affordable tool in cancer detection and diagnostics. They are an improvement over surgical biopsies as they allow multiple samples to be taken over time with simple noninvasive tests. Liquid biopsies are performed on body fluids to look for cancer cells, fragments of circulating tumor DNA, RNA, and specific proteins. Evidence of these biomarkers provides insight about tumor burden, disease progression, and metastasis. Biomarkers can reveal genetic patterns, mutations, protein expressions, or metabolic changes in the cancer cells, which can help predict potential tumor behaviors and treatment targets.

Next-generation sequencing is helping detect even very low levels of biomarkers. As more tests are developed for other body fluids like urine, saliva, and cerebrospinal fluid, the accuracy of the biopsies will improve as well. And as genetic sequencing becomes faster and cheaper, liquid biopsies could become a standard tool in early diagnosis, treatment selection, and real-time disease monitoring.

In the future, the hope is that these tests will become increasingly sensitive and specific, and that they will be able to find cancer before it becomes clinically detectable. Some multi-cancer early detection (MCED) tests already exist, and more are being developed and assessed, offering the potential to screen for cancers that currently do not yet have effective screening tests, such as ovarian and pancreatic cancer.

Liquid biopsies also have the potential to find residual cancer cells after treatment, thereby addressing cancer recurrence as early as possible. Synthetic biopsies are an emerging early detection technology that uses bioengineered DNA to force cancer cells to produce more biomarkers, making the presence of tumors more obvious. This technology has the potential to find tumors before they become clinically detectable. The National Cancer Institute's Early Detection Research Network (EDRN) is a consortium of academic and private sector investigators who are focused on the discovery of new biomarkers and imaging methods for early cancer detection and risk assessment. One of its goals is to find biomarkers that could distinguish aggressive early-stage cancers from slow-growing ones, which would help prevent overtreatment.

New biomarkers and pathways are being identified thanks to the fields of proteomics (the study of proteins) and metabolomics (the study of metabolites). All of these biomarkers help create a comprehensive picture of an individual patient's cancer, not only at the time of diagnosis, but throughout treatment, allowing therapies to be modified based on changes in the cancer itself. This will also help reveal how cancers develop resistance under treatment pressure. As the field of precision medicine becomes more accurate and accessible, an increasing variety of biomarkers will be integrated into clinical guidelines.

Scientists are discovering more about the tumor microenvironment and how the tumor relies on specific metabolic pathways to grow. Identifying those pathways will lead to therapies that can target and block them, effectively starving the cancer cells. And while most current targeted therapies focus on driver mutations, the mutations that directly contribute to cancer development and progression, future research in genomics will explore the role of passenger mutations. Passenger mutations represent the majority of mutations in cancer cells, they are "silent" and seem to have little to no impact on cancer development. But recent research suggests that passenger mutations are not always neutral mutations after all, and could, in some instances, be capable of destabilizing cancer progression. Drugs targeting this are still in early-stage research, but ultimately, exploiting passenger mutations could hold the key for future therapies.

Cancer stem cells have also become the focus of research into the tumor microenvironment due to their unique properties. These cells have the same characteristics as normal stem cells, including self-renewal and the ability to differentiate into other cell types. Cancer stem cells, which are involved in the initiation, progression, and recurrence of many cancers, support tumor growth and contribute to treatment resistance. Research is currently investigating ways to target these cells and inhibit their behavior in the hope that metastasis and recurrence could be suppressed. Developing therapies that target cancer stem cell markers would also enhance current treatments by shrinking the cancer stem cell population within the tumor.

Spatial biology is an emerging field that is expanding the scope of precision medicine. Spatial biology is the study of the way molecules, cells, and tissues are organized and interact in their natural environment, how cells fit within the context of tissue, and what the environment says about their behavior. It looks at the architecture of the tissue and maps cellular pathways in both two and three dimensions, which allows researchers to see molecular changes in tumors cell by cell.

Usually, cancer cells are studied in isolation, by dissolving tissue and culturing cells, techniques which remove the sample from the context of its environment. The tumor microenvironment and tumor heterogeneity have long been considered significant obstacles to cancer treatment because they are complex and dynamic. Spatial biology is beginning to demonstrate this complexity by mapping tumors at the molecular level while maintaining their spatial arrangement, and by tracking their interactions with the immune system.

The field takes advantage of many advanced technologies. Spatial transcriptomics and epigenomics, which map gene activity and expression, help researchers better understand cellular interactions. Imaging-based technologies play a significant role in being able to analyze how cells and their components relate to one another. Multiplexed imaging is an emerging technology that works by labeling and visualizing many biological markers at the same time on a single tissue sample. Different dyes, antibodies, or "tags" are applied to highlight specific proteins, RNA, or cell structures, all while preserving the tissue's architecture. Some of these techniques include immunofluorescence and mass-spectrometry-based imaging.

This massive amount of new information is helping researchers understand the biological processes that influence a tumor's response to therapy, to find the weak points in the cancer, and to develop effective strategies to target them. Spatial biology can potentially be used to identify new drug targets and create more personalized treatments based on each tumor's unique spatial characteristics.

All of the data generated by the study of spatial biology requires specialized computer programs, algorithms, databases, and data management tools to help researchers process and interpret the huge amount of information they collect. This makes it possible to identify patterns and draw conclusions. Many of the tools used in spatial biology use artificial intelligence (AI) techniques like graph-based approaches and machine learning. And as the field grows, there will be an increased need for AI tools to support it.

AI and computational oncology are the future of cancer research because of the sheer breadth and diversity of information that is being collected. They are revolutionizing the field by helping to transform the data into insights. AI is driven by computer algorithms that can quickly aggregate and detect patterns in large amounts of data, a skill that would take the human brain far more time and effort. AI has the potential to be used not only for studying the mechanisms of cancer, but also in cancer detection and diagnostics, predicting molecular targets for new drugs, creating simulations for understanding tumor behavior, and improving cancer surveillance and care. These approaches are leading to more precise, personalized cancer therapies.

According to scientists at the University of Hawaii Cancer Center, AI can detect subtle changes in medical scans, up to 65,000 shades of gray while the human eye can distinguish at most 256. This precision helps detect very early signs of cancer, improving accuracy in screenings. And the speed at which the AI can read images could not only free radiologists to devote more time to analyzing suspicious images but also enable more patients to access screening.

In 2023, MIT announced the development of an AI model called "Sybil" that can predict lung cancer up to six years in advance using a single low-dose CT scan. The Food and Drug Administration (FDA) has already approved several AI products to detect cancer from mammograms, and authorized the marketing of AI to help pathologists identify prostate cancer. These kinds of readings are not yet covered by insurance, however, and they can increase the risk of overdiagnosis and overtreatment. The goal for future research into AI-powered diagnostics is to demonstrate a clear benefit in patient outcomes.

AI and augmented reality (AR) are increasingly demonstrating how they can improve surgical planning and execution by offering surgeons enhanced visualization and decision-making tools. AI driven robotic surgery has the potential to increase accuracy and improve recovery time. AI can analyze and enhance imaging data to predict outcomes and inform surgical strategies in real time.

AR allows for the overlay of digital information during a procedure. Not only does this offer surgeons the opportunity to practice techniques in a virtual environment, it can also enhance navigation, visibility, and decision-making during live surgery, thereby minimizing damage to surrounding tissue. The use of these technologies is already being applied in orthopedic, trauma, and spinal surgery.

Aside from managing the data generated by research fields like spatial biology, AI can create predictive models to develop computer simulations. These simulations can be used to predict how a cancer might progress, anticipate interactions, create personalized treatments, and forecast possible outcomes for individual patients. At the National Cancer Institute (NCI), researchers are using AI to anticipate how T-cells respond to tumors, and are developing predictive models to map common drug pathways and survival outcomes.

In a collaboration between NCI and the Department of Energy, a program called Modeling Outcomes Using Surveillance Data and Scalable Artificial Intelligence for Cancer (MOSSAIC) has scientists using AI to feed data into the NCI Surveillance, Epidemiology, and End Results (SEER) program more quickly, and are developing algorithms to pull information back out more efficiently, saving thousands of hours of time.

One of the major challenges with these models is the difficulty in accessing detailed information. Big data integration is needed to manage the enormous volume and variety of data from multiple fields such as genomics, proteomics, transcriptomics, and metabolomics (also called multi-omics). The NCI's Cancer Moonshot Biobank is a longitudinal study collecting biological specimens and data from an ethnically and geographically diverse population of cancer patients throughout their treatment. It is designed to be used with machine learning to accelerate cancer research and further understand the complexities of cancer biology. Large projects around the world, like The Cancer Genome Atlas in the United States and the Catalogue of Somatic Mutations in Cancer (COSMIC) in the UK, have now determined the genome sequences of thousands of cancer samples. Most importantly, these and other initiatives facilitate data sharing among researchers, and they play an important role in driving computational oncology by providing real-world patient data.

But new technology does not come without its ethical questions and limitations. Predictive or simulated personalized treatment plans must be based on integrated patient data, and personal data privacy and security concerns are more significant than ever. There are also concerns over what use insurance providers would make of this technology in determining the cost of coverage. Regulation and compliance will have to catch up with the various new ways data will be used.

And AI is only as effective as the data it is trained on, data which is collected and entered by a human being who has the potential to be fallible or malicious. The medical community is still far from the mass adoption of these technologies, partly because they may not yet be as reliable or unbiased as they need to be. In addition, should the AI be wrong, malpractice and liability issues will have to be addressed.

The bottom line is that although AI has the potential of being a revolutionary research tool, the algorithm does not replace the researcher or physician. It should be used to enhance their skills and judgment. It should not validate its own results or make decisions. But it does have the potential to increase the speed, accuracy, and accessibility of cancer care in the future. The integration of AI into cancer care reflects an important trend toward more data-driven approaches in oncology and precision medicine.

The microbiome and its role in cancer have received increasing attention in recent years. The microbiome refers to the massive community of microorganisms that live on and in the human body, particularly the gut. It is a complex and dynamic ecosystem that contributes to how well our bodies function and influences our health. The gut is especially rich in species, and these microorganisms are necessary for healthy digestion, immune function, and the synthesis of vitamins. An imbalance in the microbiome, called dysbiosis, can be caused by things like frequent antibiotic use, diet, and gastrointestinal tract infections, and it can allow bacteria and toxins to leak through the intestinal lining. Dysbiosis can cause certain microorganisms to produce toxins and alter the functions of the immune system which can lead to inflammatory diseases, metabolic disorders, and some cancers.

Recent studies have shown how the microbiome influences not only the development of certain types of cancer but also how the composition of the microbiome can influence the body's reaction to drugs. The fact that certain microorganisms could enhance or diminish the effectiveness of cancer therapies makes it a very relevant area of study, and there is a growing interest to see how specific populations can be exploited to improve cancer outcomes.

These bacteria, viruses, and fungi number in the trillions, and each type has unique genetic material. With recent advances in genomics and sequencing, there is growing interest in personalized microbiome-based treatments to restore a healthy gut balance, improving immune responses, enhancing treatment effectiveness, and reducing side effects. In addition, incorporating microbiome profiling into the patient's personalized medical record could help identify which individuals are more or less likely to benefit from specific therapies. A deeper understanding of the microbiome's characteristics and functions could lead to more effective and personalized cancer care.

So, is the future of cancer research bright? The broad technologies which are driving the direction of cancer research certainly represent the foundation for future breakthroughs, and there is no shortage of avenues to explore. We are getting better at treating cancer. We are closer to making cancer a manageable, if not curable, disease. We are also making great strides in preventing it, which is ultimately the best and most cost-effective approach. While challenges remain, the current momentum of scientific innovations and breakthroughs is only accelerating.

Case Studies

Case 1. Talia's Colon Cancer Story

Talia is a 41-year-old woman, and an active and health-conscious professional. She works at a desk but exercises, maintains a fairly balanced diet, and consumes little alcohol. She begins experiencing abdominal cramping. It does not interfere much with her life, but it is persistent. She also notices changes in bowel habits. She assumes it is stress, related to her high-pressure job. When the discomfort turns into pain, she goes to the emergency room. The doctor there suspects it may be related to her menstrual cycle, or irritable bowel syndrome. She remains concerned, however, as she is now seeing blood in her stool. She follows up with her primary care physician because she now feels she needs a colonoscopy. Her doctor is reluctant, she is young and has no significant family history of cancer, so he recommends noninvasive blood and stool tests instead. After further discussion, and some strong advocacy on Talia's part, he orders a colonoscopy. The results reveal that Talia has colon cancer. She is in shock. She does not understand how this is possible, she feels she is too young to have cancer, she is not even old enough to be screened for colorectal cancer. She tests negative for any hereditary mutations, and she does not seem to have any significant environmental or lifestyle risk factors.

Talia undergoes surgery to remove the tumor in her colon, an approach that seems initially successful. But follow-up scans later detect a single metastasis in her liver. At this point, Talia falls apart. Not only does she have a disease that should only happen to old people, but it is advanced, it has evidently been developing for a long time inside her without her ever suspecting. Given the advanced stage of her cancer, Talia's medical team puts together a personalized treatment plan that is both aggressive and mindful of the fact that she is still relatively young. The overall goal is to maximize long-term control over the disease while preserving her quality of life.

She receives a combination of chemotherapy and targeted therapy infusions. She is healthy and she copes pretty well with the side effects of chemotherapy. She does lose weight as her appetite decreases. The chemo makes her food taste bad. The upside for her is that she is forced to slow down and focus on lowering her stress and improving her nutrition and sleep habits.

Her cancer responds well to the treatment and her medical team decides to address the liver metastasis with radiofrequency ablation, a minimally invasive procedure that uses heat to destroy the lesion. Genetic profiling of her tumor reveals Talia has a mutation which is only found in about 5 percent of metastatic colorectal cancer. This mutation makes her a candidate for an immunotherapy drug called a checkpoint inhibitor. Where chemotherapy slows the cancer's growth, immunotherapy will help her immune system to fight the cancer.

With this personalized combination of therapies, Talia is not in complete remission, but the disease is stabilized. She is closely monitored with imaging and lab work, and she adapts to living with certain side effects like fatigue and neuropathy in her hands and feet. She remains on maintenance therapy which allows her to live with her cancer as a manageable chronic condition.

Analysis

Talia's case reflects the growing incidence of early-onset colorectal cancer. The exact causes are still unclear, but researchers suspect a variety of lifestyle and dietary factors like obesity, sedentary lifestyles, ultra-processed foods, and changes in the gut microbiome. As a result, the American Cancer Society has recently updated its guidelines for colorectal cancer screening, lowering the recommended age to forty-five. The fact that she is still younger than the recommended screening guidelines highlights the need for education and awareness beyond traditional high-risk groups. This is crucial because young people are more likely to delay diagnosis. They may be unaware of what their symptoms represent, or they believe they are not old enough to be concerned about cancer. And their physicians are certainly not expecting that kind of diagnosis either. The result is that their cancer tends to go undetected for longer, and when it is found, it is more advanced.

Luckily, Talia also knows her body and trusts her instincts, so she advocates for herself when her symptoms are dismissed, and she pushes for diagnostic testing. Some symptoms should never be ignored, regardless of age or perceived health, and providers should take patient concerns seriously, even when they fall outside statistical norms. This is especially true with conditions for which early intervention is critical.

Talia's case also reflects the shift toward personalized cancer medicine, where a variety of treatments are administered alongside one another. Combining standard and personalized approaches has been shown to improve outcomes. Genetic testing plays a role in Talia's care, showing how treatments can be tailored to the unique biology of the patient.

And although the recent increase in cancer incidence among younger people is still unexplained, we are seeing people living with cancer much longer than ever before. Talia's experience reflects a broader trend of patients not only living longer after their diagnosis but also maintaining a sense of normalcy and quality of life.

Case 2. Lucas's Hodgkin Lymphoma Story

Lucas is a fourteen-year-old boy who has just started high school. His parents have noticed lately he has no energy and seems drained. After going to the doctor with a fever and swollen glands, he is prescribed antibiotics. The swelling persists, and after some weeks of increasing fatigue and unexplained weight loss, he is referred for testing and imaging. A biopsy reveals he has Hodgkin lymphoma. Scans show the lymph nodes in his chest and abdomen are also affected, but his organs and bone marrow are still clear. His Hodgkin lymphoma is stage III.

Lucas is torn between denial and dread, but the treatments keep him occupied. His oncologist recommends four cycles of chemotherapy, and then, more imaging to see how things are going. He receives radiation on his chest and abdomen. Lucas and his family are counseled about the risks and side effects of his treatment, including potential future cardiovascular and fertility issues. Someone talks to him about banking sperm for the future, but he is not comfortable having that conversation. His parents are only concerned about his survival.

The chemotherapy is hard on Lucas; he stops going to school and starts taking classes online at home. He is tired all the time. Despite his anti-nausea medications, he struggles with queasiness and loses even more weight. The radiation is causing redness and sensitivity on his chest and stomach, and he is finding it hard to swallow and painful to cough. But the hardest thing for him to bear is that within the first few weeks, he loses his hair. He is bald, he has lost his eyebrows, and he feels like a freak. He feels isolated and disconnected, and he is irked by the way his family treats him. At times he feels like they do not care enough about what is happening to him, and other times he wishes they would leave him alone and stop treating him like he is helpless. Between the stress, the treatment side effects, and hormonal shifts, Lucas feels drowned by mood swings. The cancer center recommends counseling for his anxiety, and supportive care to help manage his symptoms.

Fortunately for Lucas, he is young and otherwise healthy, and responds well. After six months he reaches the end of his treatment. He successfully achieves remission. The relief is immediate. He has been told he will need to see an endocrinologist to assess his hormone levels, and he may need fertility counseling. He will need to have his heart and lung function monitored for a long time, he is at risk of developing other kinds of cancer because of the treatment he underwent, and there is a high risk of recurrence.

He is told to eat well and stay healthy, which he does, but he still feels disconnected because deep down he is petrified at the thought that the cancer will come back. Lucas starts to engage in risky behaviors like drinking and drugs. He starts drag-racing. He is into his twenties now and believes he might as well live while he can; it might all be gone tomorrow. His family is worried but unwilling to interfere. They are simply grateful he is alive.

One day Lucas realizes that he has in fact survived, and he has a real life to live. He contacts his cancer care team for advice on getting mental health counseling for cancer survivors. Beyond the long-term monitoring of his health, he admits he also needs psychosocial support. He moves forward with life. He gets married and is eager to start a family. But the consequences of the cancer begin to surface when Lucas discovers that the cumulative impact of chemotherapy and radiation may have caused him to be sterile. With his mental health under control and his experience navigating the health care system, Lucas feels he can take on this battle and starts researching his options. If he can beat cancer, he can get through anything.

Analysis

Lucas's story shows that kids get cancer too. It can be a very different experience, and one that has long-lasting implications. Luckily for him, his family and his doctor do not downplay his symptoms and move quickly to identify the lymphoma. Hodgkin lymphoma has a high survival rate, especially when caught early.

Lucas does not start off with the best prognosis, but the treatment for Hodgkin lymphoma has come a long way, and his youth improves his chances. Despite having significant short-term side effects from the treatment, it is ultimately effective. However, the long-term effects of cancer treatment can be harsh and far reaching, and the risk of infertility is a common concern for survivors of childhood and adolescent cancers. Younger people have a hard time believing bad things can happen to them. Should Lucas have banked his sperm? Was that conversation simply not a priority at the time? Sometimes it is hard to see into the future, beyond the treatment. But the better patients and their families are prepared, the better they will be able to cope. Lucas's case shows how important it is to have comprehensive survivorship care, including discussions about fertility, psychological, social, and emotional support, and long-term health monitoring.

Nowadays more attention is being paid to mental health during cancer treatment. Teenagers like Lucas face more than just medical challenges. The counseling he receives certainly helps him cope with body image changes, fear, and isolation, and gives him confidence to finish high school. But the cancer story is not over when treatment ends, and the fear of recurrence leaves its mark on Lucas. Mental health support is crucial, especially for young people who may not have developed healthy ways to cope with anxiety and stress. But like Lucas, many survivors of childhood and adolescent cancer go on to live full and meaningful lives. His experience has shown him how resilient and capable he really is, and his journey has taught him how to recognize what matters.

Case 3. Linda's Melanoma Story

Linda is a 62-year-old woman who has spent much of her life outdoors, interested in nature and spirituality. She grew up at a time when getting a sunburn simply meant getting a start on your summer tan. She evened out her deep tan by using tanning beds. She always assumed this gave her some protection against the sun, and certainly never worried about skin cancer. For years she has had unusual moles on her leg, a couple of them are dark and irregular in shape, but she has dismissed them as harmless. One day, she comments that one of the moles is scaly and bleeding and a friend urges her to go to a dermatologist, just to have them checked out. After some hesitation, she schedules an appointment.

A biopsy confirms that Linda has melanoma, and further testing shows that the cancer has spread to her lymph nodes. She is referred to an oncologist who recommends surgery to remove the melanomas, as well as the affected lymph nodes. Depending on the tissue analysis, she will be treated with immunotherapy or targeted therapy. But Linda is horrified at the thought of such invasive and toxic treatments. She tells her doctor that she knows someone who refused treatment for skin cancer and went on to live for decades. The oncologist explains that while it is true that some melanomas grow very slowly and are therefore simply monitored, her own case is aggressive and requires immediate treatment. With Linda's age and overall health, the prognosis may be poor but with current personalized therapeutic strategies, outcomes are better than they used to be.

Linda is hesitant about conventional treatments though, she prefers to wait and see, and she starts researching alternative therapies. She has always disliked the idea of putting chemicals in her body, she still feels healthy, and she is probably in a bit of denial too. She has always gravitated toward natural cures because it seems like they would be gentler, and more likely to boost her body's own healing powers. She decides to try herbal supplements, mushroom extracts, turmeric, and apricot kernels. They are marketed as having anti-cancer properties. For the same reasons, she received high-dose vitamin C infusions. She also makes dietary changes which involve juicing and organic vegetarian meals. Linda schedules regular energy healing and acupuncture sessions.

Her doctor urges her to trust proven treatments and suggests using some of these complementary therapies alongside conventional ones. But she also assures Linda that the decision is hers. Her friend tells her she is crazy, that she is betting her life on something she has seen on the internet and just because a treatment is natural does not mean it is safe. But ultimately, the riskiest thing Linda is doing is delaying a proven and effective treatment.

Within a few months, Linda notices new symptoms, like fatigue and unexplained weight loss. Her lymph nodes are swollen, and she returns to her doctor. She learns that the cancer has spread beyond her lymph nodes and that curative treatment may no longer be an option. The doctor's focus shifts to palliative care and maintaining quality of life. She urges Linda to maintain some of her alternative treatments. Her natural organic diet is certainly good for her, and her mind-body therapies like energy healing and acupuncture are going to support her emotional and psychological wellbeing. She cautions her about supplements to make sure nothing is interacting with drugs she might need for pain or symptom control. And she says Linda might even receive palliative radiation if the tumors begin causing discomfort from growth, obstruction, or bleeding. Aside from alleviating symptoms, this kind of radiation may also extend survival.

Linda goes through a rough emotional time, she feels guilty, cheated, helpless, and unable to process her experience. But out of this turmoil, Linda finds some inner strength and a new appreciation for the life she has left. She stood by her beliefs. Some days are better than others, but she now feels a deeper understanding of faith and spirituality.

Analysis

Linda grew up during a time when people did not realize the danger of serious sunburn, and her assumption that her suntan would confer some kind of protection from cancer was wrong. Even though anyone with deep toned or tanned skin may be, statistically, slightly less likely to get skin cancer, they should always get any unusual moles checked. The fact that years went by before she got her moles examined means her cancer is far more advanced and she has far fewer options.

Not all skin cancers are localized and slow growing. Melanoma in particular can be aggressive and unpredictable, which is why early detection and treatment are so important. This is also why delaying conventional therapy can reduce the chance of survival. With aggressive cancer especially, patient education and timely intervention are crucial. Linda's doctor has certainly seen enough cases to know when something is urgent, but she lets her know the choice is hers.

People sometimes have very strong feelings about the medical field, drugs, and doctors. They may have an affinity for natural or holistic medicine. Linda is also in denial and looking for some kind of autonomy in the face of her fear. The alternative therapies she gravitates toward might have been safe and helpful when used alongside conventional therapy, but there simply is not enough evidence to show they can be used effectively in its place. Ultimately, it is difficult to tell how much longer Linda would have survived with conventional therapy, or whether she would have been as satisfied with her quality of life. Treatment decisions can be intensely personal and cancer patients should be able to navigate their cancer journey on their own terms. They need to know what gives them the best possible chance based on available information, and they need to trust that their choices will be respected.

Case 4. Renee's Cervical Cancer Story

Renee is a 35-year-old woman and mother of two. She is a bit overweight, but she works in the service industry and is on her feet a lot. And since she started raising her children, she realizes how important it is for her to take care of her health, so she recently quit smoking. She goes in for a routine pelvic exam at a community health clinic, even though she has no symptoms and wants to skip the appointment due to her long shifts and inadequate health insurance. Her provider is concerned by something he sees during the exam. The Pap smear and HPV test confirm the presence of squamous cell carcinoma of the cervix.

Renee is shocked by the diagnosis, and a little put off when the provider tells her that the cancer was probably caused by a human papillomavirus (HPV) infection and because she was a smoker. The way he tells her seems to imply it was somehow her fault. He is rushed and abrupt, and she is left with a few pamphlets about treatment and co-pay assistance, which she barely has the focus to read. She goes home feeling devastated, confused, and alone. She does not even tell her family until a couple of weeks have gone by. After finding the entire experience frightening as well as embarrassing, she feels like she has no faith in this provider, or this community health clinic. And even though the cost of medical care weighs on her mind she insists on a second opinion.

She begins by looking at the National Cancer Institute (NCI) website. It shows her a list of facilities nearby that offer expert treatment as well as financial assistance. She calls one of the cancer centers, and their financial services department helps her navigate her options given the fact that she has limited insurance. A financial counselor finds her treatment assistance through the National Breast and Cervical Cancer Early Detection Program.

The care team at the cancer center confirms the diagnosis of early-stage cervical cancer. They tell her that it is true her cancer was probably caused by an HPV infection, an infection she was probably never even aware of. And this is significant because there is now a vaccine that can potentially prevent this type of cancer. They tell her that her past smoking may also have contributed to her cancer, but by quitting she is already improving her health immeasurably. She finds the people she is dealing with supportive and empowering. The provider she is seeing now is positive, focused on her as a person, and engaged in the process. Renee feels confident she can undergo the treatment.

Her cervical cancer is Stage I, her tumor is about the size of a peanut. She opts for a hysterectomy, in which the uterus and cervix, as well as nearby lymph nodes are removed. She already has two children, so the loss of her fertility is less important to her than being certain all of the cancer is gone. Also, because she is generally healthy, she has a good chance of recovering quickly from surgery. The care team explains that if her lymph nodes are clear after her hysterectomy, and there is no evidence of spread beyond the cervix, she likely will not need radiation or chemotherapy. This turns out to be the case, to her immense relief. Thanks to early detection, her treatment is successful, and she is told her prognosis is excellent.

Renee is now cancer-free and has become a strong advocate for routine cervical cancer screenings, especially advocating for the uninsured or underinsured. And knowing that a simple HPV vaccination can prevent this kind of cancer, she makes a commitment to have her children vaccinated when they reach the appropriate age.

Analysis

When diagnosed at an early stage, the five-year survival rate for cervical cancer is over 90 percent, so Renee is wise to have kept her appointment for a routine screening. Even when there are no symptoms, screening and early detection can save lives.

Renee's experience with her first provider is unfortunate. Between being understaffed and underfunded, the community clinic is unable to really spend the time with her that she needs. And the fact that she senses friction with the provider makes the whole experience even worse than it already is. It is perfectly fine, and even essential sometimes, to seek a second opinion. Renee now feels she has more control over her health decisions, and a better understanding of her diagnosis and treatment plan because of it. It is also important for Renee to find a care team that is respectful and supportive. Once she feels heard, she becomes more proactive, optimistic, and trustful. She acknowledges that she wants a provider and a team that treats her more like a partner than a patient, and whom she believes is on her side. She learns that it is OK to want that.

Renee discovers that many cancer centers and nonprofit organizations offer help, not only with treatment but also screenings, transportation, childcare, and medication. Once she is no longer worried about costs, she is able to focus on healing. Her interaction with patient advocates who guide her through paperwork, insurance issues, and general decision-making, teaches her that patients do better when they speak up for their needs and ask questions. She becomes an advocate herself, helping people who are in the same situation. Renee now also has a real appreciation for cancer awareness and education. Understanding what caused her cancer and how it is now practically preventable thanks to a vaccine, empowers her to protect her children and share what she knows. Through her advocacy work, she wants future patients to feel educated and supported, and to be able to access the best care available.

Case 5. Max's Glioblastoma Story

Max is a 28-year-old graphic designer and fitness buff. He begins experiencing headaches, and double vision. He assumes it is overwork, or maybe he just needs new contact lenses. One morning, while he is out running, he experiences a seizure and is rushed to the emergency room. He is given a neurological exam, and an MRI reveals he has a mass in his brain. It is glioblastoma, an aggressive and often fatal brain tumor.

Max is stunned. He is young, healthy, and active; he has never had a day's illness in his life. He tells his partner this cannot be happening, that there has been a mistake. He keeps feeling like this is happening to someone else, not him. He cycles through disbelief, denial, fear, and anger.

Max's prognosis is poor. Even with treatment, the average survival time for someone with glioblastoma is 12–18 months. His medical team have told him that his youth and good health might give him a better chance than older patients, but the tumor is aggressive and there is a high likelihood of recurrence. They are honest and realistic about this. They also emphasize the importance of managing his symptoms and quality of life with palliative care from the outset.

His tumor is located in a part of the brain that makes surgery more complicated, but he undergoes a craniotomy to remove as much of it as possible. The surgery is followed by six weeks of daily radiation combined with oral chemotherapy. Max is given medications to control his seizures, steroids to reduce brain swelling, and a variety of drugs to help with headaches. His doctors advise supportive care like physical and occupational therapy to help him regain strength and balance.

He wakes up every morning and for just a split second, he has forgotten he has brain cancer. But then he remembers, and he feels oppressive fear and sadness. Max's mental health fluctuates between feeling determined and hopeful, and feeling depressed and mad at God. He tries to maintain a journal about his experience, hoping it will help him process his feelings. But he is also facing cognitive changes and mood swings. Max feels guilty about putting his family and friends through so much pain, but at the same time he finds it hard to talk to them. He joins a support group for young adults with cancer which helps a great deal because they "get it."

Eight months after his initial diagnosis, Max has a follow-up scan which shows tumor progression. His oncologist gives him his options: he can try a different kind of chemotherapy which may have stronger side effects, he can join a clinical trial for an immunotherapy drug, or he can cut back his treatment to supportive care only. He is exhausted, but he decides on the trial, thinking that at the very least he will contribute to research even if the benefit to him is limited. The experimental treatment causes additional fatigue, nausea, and worsens his brain fog. Despite his anti-epileptic medication, Max starts having more seizures.

His visits with the palliative care team become more frequent; they are managing his symptoms with medications and supportive therapies. He is taking low-dose opioids for pain. They refer him to a social worker to help him navigate his end-of-life and advance care planning. He tries to resist thinking about those things, but he is too exhausted to argue. Once he begins, he realizes that making his end-of-life plans actually gives him a purpose.

Max's outlook begins to change, he tells himself he is not giving up, he is simply choosing a different kind of fight. He decides to stop active treatment and focus on his quality of life. He and his partner move in with his parents where he receives home hospice care. With the support of his family and the help of the hospice nurses, Max is kept comfortable and able to appreciate small moments like cuddling his dog, looking at the moon at night, and sitting quietly with his loved ones. He spends time writing letters and recording messages for his friends and his siblings. He finds a new plane of acceptance and it gives him clarity and peace. Max passes away peacefully with his family at his side, he has lived his final months on his own terms.

Analysis

Max's experience highlights the emotional and physical toll of cancer, as well as the reality that sometimes the disease is simply incurable. He sees that supportive care like palliative care, group support, and mental health counseling help him live and cope better. He has unique challenges because he is so young and fewer than 5 percent of patients with glioblastoma survive beyond five years. The support he gets while he navigates the emotional and existential impact of a terminal diagnosis makes all the difference. Max grieves for himself, his future plans and dreams, but he also finds he has meaningful life left to live.

Participating in a clinical trial gives Max a sense that he is contributing, which is powerful. But his decision to stop aggressive therapy is also powerful. The benefits no longer outweigh the burden. Patients have the right to choose how they want to spend the time they have left, and it is OK to say "no" to more treatment.

Advance planning proves to be a gift for Max. It gives him some purpose and as he ensures his choices are respected, he is also helping to prepare his loved ones. Being proactive helps him find peace of mind so he can live the time he has with meaning, dignity, and connection.

Glossary

Ablation: A minimally invasive procedure that destroys cancerous tissue using methods like heat, cold, or chemicals.

Acute: Describes symptoms or conditions that develop rapidly and are often severe but short-lived.

Advance Care Planning: The process of discussing and documenting the patient's choices concerning medical and end-of-life care.

Alternative Medicine: Treatments used instead of conventional medicine, often lacking scientific validation and potentially risky if used as the sole treatment.

Artificial Intelligence (AI): Machines or software that can process and analyze large sets of data to support cancer research and diagnostics by identifying patterns and solving problems.

Benign: Refers to tumors that are non-cancerous and do not spread to other parts of the body.

Biomarkers: Biological molecules found in blood, tissue, or other body fluids, that act as measurable indicators of normal or abnormal processes, which are used to track the presence or progression of a disease like cancer.

Biopsy: The removal of a small sample of tissue for examination under a microscope, or with genetic and molecular testing, to diagnose diseases.

Cancer Recurrence: The return of cancer after a period of remission.

Carcinogen: A substance or agent capable of causing cancer by altering cellular metabolism or damaging DNA.

Carcinoma: A type of cancer that starts in epithelial cells, cells of the skin or the tissues lining internal organs.

Chemotherapy: A type of cancer treatment that uses drugs to destroy rapidly dividing cancer cells.

Chronic: A term used to describe conditions or symptoms that persist over a long period of time, often for months or years.

Complementary Medicine: Therapies used in addition to conventional treatments, such as acupuncture or nutritional support.

Diagnosis: The process of identifying a disease or condition from its signs, symptoms, and test results.

Endoscopy: A procedure during which a flexible tube with a light and camera is used to view internal parts of the body and sometimes deliver therapy.

Gene Editing: The process of altering DNA sequences in living cells, potentially to correct mutations or enhance treatments.

Genomics: The study of the genome, including the structure, function, evolution, and mapping of genes.

Hospice Care: Specialized care focusing on quality of life and comfort when curative treatments are no longer effective.

Imaging: Techniques like MRI, CT, and PET scans used to visualize structures inside the body.

Immune System: The body's defense system against infections and diseases, including cancer.

Immunotherapy: Treatments that stimulate or restore the immune system's ability to fight cancer.

Integrative Medicine: A comprehensive approach that combines conventional medical treatments with complementary therapies.

Invasive: Refers to cancer that has spread beyond the original tissue into surrounding areas.

Leukemia: A type of cancer that starts in blood-forming tissue such as bone marrow.

Liquid Biopsy: A non-invasive test that detects cancer-related genetic material in fluids like blood.

Lymphatic System: A network of tissues and organs that help rid the body of toxins and waste, and plays a role in cancer spread.

Lymphoma: A type of cancer that begins in the lymphatic system, typically in lymph nodes.

Malignant: Describes cancerous tumors that can invade and destroy nearby tissue and spread to other parts of the body.

Metastasis: The spread of cancer cells from the original tumor to other parts of the body.

Mutation: A change in the DNA sequence that can lead to disease, including cancer.

Next-Generation Sequencing: A fast and efficient method to sequence DNA, used for analyzing cancer-related mutations.

Oncology: The study and treatment of cancer.

Palliative Care: Care that focuses on relieving symptoms and improving quality of life for patients with serious illness.

Pathology: The study of body tissues, cells, and fluids, to diagnose diseases and examine their causes, development, and effects on the body.

Personalized or Precision Medicine: A treatment strategy tailored to the individual characteristics of each patient and their disease. An approach to patient care that considers individual variability in genes, environment, and lifestyle.

Photodynamic Therapy: A cancer treatment that uses a photosensitizing drug activated by light to destroy cancer cells.

Prognosis: The predicted course and outcome of a disease.

Radiation Therapy: A treatment that uses high-energy radiation to kill or shrink cancer cells.

Reactive Oxygen Species (ROS): Highly reactive molecules that are a byproduct of cellular metabolism. Their function is to act as messengers in a variety of normal biological processes; however, when present in excess, they cause cellular damage and contribute to disease.

Remission: A period during which the signs and symptoms of cancer are reduced or disappear.

Risk Factor: Any attribute, characteristic, or exposure that increases the likelihood of developing a disease.

Sarcoma: A type of cancer that begins in the bones or soft tissues like fat, muscles, or blood vessels.

Secondary Cancer: Also known as metastatic cancer, a cancer that has spread from its original, or primary, site to another part of the body.

Targeted Therapy: Drugs or other treatments that block the growth of cancer by interfering with specific molecules.

Tumor: An abnormal mass of tissue that may be benign or malignant.

Tumor-Agnostic Therapy: A treatment that targets a specific genetic mutation in cancer, regardless of cancer type.

Tumor Heterogeneity: The existence of different types of cancer cells within the same tumor.

Tumor Microenvironment: The surrounding cells and structures that influence the behavior and treatment of a tumor.

Tumor Profiling: Analyzing the genetic and molecular characteristics of a tumor to guide treatment.

Directory of Resources

Organizations

American Cancer Society (ACS)
https://www.cancer.org
The ACS is a nationwide voluntary health organization dedicated to eliminating cancer. It funds research, provides patient support, and promotes cancer prevention and education.

American Cancer Society Cancer Action Network (ACS CAN)
https://www.fightcancer.org/
ACS CAN is the advocacy affiliate of the American Cancer Society. It works to make cancer a national priority by influencing public policies at the federal, state, and local levels to promote cancer prevention, funding, research, and access to care.

Cancer Grand Challenges
https://www.cancergrandchallenges.org/
Cancer Grand Challenges is a global funding initiative co-founded by Cancer Research UK and the National Cancer Institute (NCI). It supports interdisciplinary research teams working to solve some of the biggest challenges in cancer research.

Centers for Disease Control and Prevention (CDC)
https://www.cdc.gov
The CDC is the United States' national public health agency. It conducts critical science and provides health information to protect against health threats and respond to outbreaks and emergencies.

Environmental Protection Agency (EPA)
https://www.epa.gov
The EPA protects human health and the environment by enforcing regulations on air, water, and soil pollutants.

Food and Drug Administration (FDA)
https://www.fda.gov
The FDA is a US federal agency responsible for protecting public health by ensuring the safety, efficacy, and security of drugs, biological products, and medical devices. It also regulates dietary supplements, food safety, cosmetics, and tobacco products.

National Cancer Institute (NCI)
https://www.cancer.gov
Part of the NIH, the NCI leads national efforts in cancer research and training. It provides funding, clinical trial information, and public education on cancer detection, prevention, and treatment.

National Institutes of Health (NIH)
https://www.nih.gov
The NIH is the primary federal agency for conducting and supporting medical research. It comprises twenty-seven institutes and centers and funds scientific studies across all aspects of health and disease.

Quackwatch
https://www.quackwatch.org
A website that monitors health frauds, myths, fads, and medical misinformation. It provides consumer protection by debunking unscientific claims.

World Health Organization (WHO)
https://www.who.int/emergencies/disease-outbreak-news
WHO is the United Nations agency responsible for coordinating international public health emergencies. It represents the public health interests of 196 member nations.

Books

Compton, Carolyn. *Cancer: The Enemy Within. A Comprehensive Textbook of Cancer's Causes, Complexities, and Consequences.* Oxford: Oxford University Press, 2020.

Nedu. *Biology Made Easy: An Illustrated Study Guide for Students to Easily Understand Cellular & Molecular Biology.* [United States]: NEDU LLC, 2021.

Stegall, Jonathan. *Cancer Secrets: An Integrative Oncologist Reveals How to Fight Cancer Using the Best of Modern Medicine and Natural Therapies.* 2nd ed. Cumming, GA: Integrative Cancer Centers of America, 2021.

Websites

PubMed
https://pubmed.ncbi.nlm.nih.gov/
A free resource developed and maintained by the National Center for Biotechnology Information (NCBI) that provides access to references and abstracts on life sciences and biomedical topics from MEDLINE and other sources.

Science Direct

https://www.sciencedirect.com/

A leading full-text scientific database offering articles and book chapters from more than 2,500 peer-reviewed journals and more than 11,000 books covering a wide range of scientific disciplines.

Index

About the Author

Lara Thompson is a freelance writer, wife, and mother, with a background in journalism. She is an independent researcher and a contributing author to ABC-CLIO's suite of electronic databases, now part of Bloomsbury Digital Resources (BDR), covering topics like Corporate Espionage, Internet Safety, Cybercrime, Consumer Fraud, Cutting and Self-Harm, as well as biographies of world leaders. This is the first publication she has written that will have a cover, which is an exciting milestone for someone who enjoys writing to enlighten and entertain.